THE HANDBOOK OF FIVE ELEMENT PRACTICE

by the same author

Keepers of the Soul
The Five Guardian Elements of Acupuncture
ISBN 978 1 84819 185 3
eISBN 978 0 85701 146 6

Patterns of Practice
Mastering the Art of Five Element Acupuncture
ISBN 978 1 84819 187 7
eISBN 978 0 85701 148 0

The Simple Guide to Five Element Acupuncture
ISBN 978 1 84819 186 0
eISBN 978 0 85701 147 3

THE HANDBOOK OF
FIVE ELEMENT PRACTICE

NORA FRANGLEN

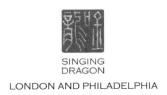

SINGING DRAGON

LONDON AND PHILADELPHIA

This edition published in 2014
by Singing Dragon
an imprint of Jessica Kingsley Publishers
73 Collier Street
London N1 9BE, UK
and
400 Market Street, Suite 400
Philadelphia, PA 19106, USA

www.singingdragon.com

First edition published by the School of Five Element Acupuncture, 2004

Copyright © Nora Franglen 2004, 2009, 2014
Cover image copyright © Hamish Horsley 2014

Front cover image: The Li River at Guilin, Southern China by Hamish Horsley. Reproduced by kind permission of the photographer.

All rights reserved. No part of this publication may be reproduced in any material form (including photocopying or storing it in any medium by electronic means and whether or not transiently or incidentally to some other use of this publication) without the written permission of the copyright owner except in accordance with the provisions of the Copyright, Designs and Patents Act 1988 or under the terms of a licence issued by the Copyright Licensing Agency Ltd, Saffron House, 6–10 Kirby Street, London EC1N 8TS. Applications for the copyright owner's written permission to reproduce any part of this publication should be addressed to the publisher.

Warning: The doing of an unauthorized act in relation to a copyright work may result in both a civil claim for damages and criminal prosecution.

Library of Congress Cataloging in Publication Data
Franglen, Nora.
  The handbook of five element practice / Nora Franglen. -- Revised.
     pages cm
  Originally published: London : School of Five Element Acupuncture, 2004.
  Includes bibliographical references and index.
  ISBN 978-1-84819-188-4 (alk. paper)
 1. Acupuncture. 2. Five agents (Chinese philosophy) I. Title.
 RM184.F58618 2014
 615.8'92--dc23
                              2013024600

British Library Cataloguing in Publication Data
A CIP catalogue record for this book is available from the British Library

ISBN 978 1 84819 188 4
eISBN 978 0 85701 145 9

Printed and bound in Great Britain

For my family

'I have read the sacred book (of the origin of the universe). It states that in the vast void of the universe exists the primordial origin of life. The five elemental phases follow the cycles of heaven and combine with the six original cosmic energies that encompass and embrace the entire universe. They set the rhythm for the growth, development, maturation, and death of all things.'

The Yellow Emperor's Classic of Medicine, tr Maoshing Ni (1995), Shambhala, Boston and London, p.236

Contents

ABOUT THE AUTHOR	11
ACKNOWLEDGEMENTS	13
Introduction	15
1. The Five Elements	17
The guardian element	19
2. Wood, Fire, Earth, Metal and Water	25
The five elements and their 12 officials	26
Introduction to the elements	27
The Wood element: The guardian element of hope and renewal	28
The Fire element: The guardian element of relationship	30
The Earth element: The guardian element of home and hearth	35
The Metal element: The guardian element of purity	37
The Water element: The medium of life	41
The qualities of the elements	45
3. Components of Five Element Diagnosis	47
The patient-practitioner relationship	47
The Traditional Diagnosis (TD)	48
TD checklist of questions	49
Note-taking	52
Sensory and emotional signatures	53
Training our senses	54
The level of imbalance	56
The causes of disease	57
4. Secondary Diagnostic Information	61
Pulse-taking	61
Blood pressure	65
Three jiao	65
Alarm points	67
Centre pulse	68
Akabane test	69
5. Treatment	73
The different stages of treatment	73
The spacing of treatments	75

Assessing the effects of treatment	76
The Law of Cure	81
The patient's role in treatment	82

6. Acupuncture Points — 83
Specific groups of points — 84

7. Blocks to Treatment — 91
Possession — 91
Aggressive Energy — 95
The Law of Husband-Wife — 100
Entry-Exit blocks — 102
Blocks caused by scars — 105

8. Treatment Techniques — 107
Needling techniques — 108
Moxibustion techniques — 110

9. Treatment Protocols — 115
The Law of Mother-Child and Sheng and Ke cycles — 115
Energy transfers — 115
Seasonal and daily treatment cycles — 120

10. Point Selection — 123
Guidelines for selecting points — 123
List of my favourite points for each element — 129
Example of point selection for first four treatments — 139

Postscript — 141

APPENDIX: TEACH YOURSELF MANUAL — 143

About the Author

Nora Franglen has a degree in Modern Languages from Cambridge University, and worked as a translator whilst bringing up a young family. Her own experience of five element acupuncture led her to study at the College of Traditional Acupuncture, Leamington Spa, UK, and she continued her postgraduate studies there under J.R. Worsley. She was Founder/Principal of the School of Five Element Acupuncture (SOFEA) in London from 1995–2007 and continues her teaching through her practice, through postgraduate work in the UK, Europe and China, and now through her blog, norafranglen.blogspot.com. She lives in London, UK.

Acknowledgements

As in all traditions, we learn from those who have gone before, and each generation of acupuncture practitioners owes a debt to those who taught them. Every time I lift a needle I am aware of that Assembly of Ancestors drawn towards me in that lovely point, Three Heater 7, and standing at my shoulder encouraging me. So to all the centuries of ancestors who have contributed their knowledge of the power of the points I give thanks. And in particular, during my lifetime, I owe a debt of gratitude to two teachers in particular. The first is J.R. Worsley, my own acupuncture master, who inspired me during his lifetime with his wisdom and deep understanding of the profound nature of what we practise. The second is Peter Eckman, historian of acupuncture, whose book *In the Footsteps of the Yellow Emperor* I reach for regularly to help elucidate one or other of the recurring questions about my practice, and whose contribution to my understanding underlies this book.

Introduction

I like to describe five element acupuncture as an ancient form of healing for a modern world. At a time when our attention is increasingly focused inwards towards the fulfilment of our inner needs, it adds something absolutely relevant to our endeavours to develop ourselves to our fullest potential, whilst bringing to the practice of acupuncture a deep understanding of the body within which our soul resides. At the touch of a needle it can guide both towards balance.

The branch of five element acupuncture which I practise and teach is blessedly simple and eminently practical. Blessedly, I feel, for all the deepest truths are simple, and the truth about human nature which a deep understanding of the five elements reveals to us is one such profound truth. Having studied it and practised it for more than 30 years, I cannot fault its ability to convey ultimately deeply profound concepts about the human being in such simple outlines. Its ability then to translate this understanding into sophisticated diagnostic and treatment procedures confirms for me the validity of this truth with each treatment I carry out.

And the aim of this book is to help others find their way to the heart of this simple truth, and to learn some of the methods which help us maintain such a focus in our treatments.

To practise our art to the highest level we have to steep ourselves in the elements before we can learn to understand at a deep level how each one expresses itself within us. We cannot truly know the Metal element, for example, until we have focused our treatment solely upon this element until it yields its secrets. Nor can an element show itself in all its nakedness until its needs are addressed directly through treatment and, even more importantly, through the practitioner's empathy with their patients which an understanding of the manifestations of each element makes possible. Any confusion of focus, any ambiguity of intent, will cloud the true picture, forming a screen behind which the element hides. We have to address each in turn with a purity of focus that allows them to emerge slowly into the open.

The vision of the human being which my own particular take on the five elements has vouchsafed me guides me through each minute of my practice. There are many other takes, many other approaches, all equally valid provided they base themselves upon the realities of human life and human health, and all make their own, but differing contribution to furthering our knowledge.

All are equally capable of leading a patient forwards towards balance. Here I concentrate upon one such approach, offering my own distillation of the many distillations of knowledge which countless generations of acupuncturists have passed on to me. What I have written here has been confirmed as being effective from my own practice and from that of others around me.

I intend this book to be used as a practical companion for students and practitioners to dip into to help them stimulate their thoughts, refresh their memories and strengthen the foundation of their practice.

To help those many people who have no opportunity to learn from a five element acupuncturist in the many different countries throughout the world who have shown an interest in reading my books, I have now included as an appendix to this new edition of the Handbook a self-help manual for those interested in learning more. This is primarily aimed at qualified acupuncturists, but can also be used by people who want to learn more before deciding whether they want to go on to study acupuncture.

The ideal introduction to a healing discipline such as five element acupuncture is in the form of a personal transmission from master to pupil. This was the only way people learned in the past, where the handing down of experience from one member of the family to the next was common practice. Modern forms of education, though, have increasingly emphasized the need to gather students together into classrooms, there to follow rigidly standardized courses with a ratio of one tutor to a roomful of students. It is little wonder, then, that against this backdrop of formalized learning, the transmission of many years of deeply personal experiences from a practitioner to a student is a luxury denied to all but the very lucky few, those ones who have been able to find a teacher whose teachings they admire and who lives close enough to them to be available at sufficiently regular intervals to pass on his/her knowledge.

This being so sadly the case now, and the situation being made even harder by the lack of good five element clinicians prepared to teach, I have decided to do what I can to fill a glaring gap through writing these lessons. Since I cannot single-handedly (or with just a tiny few other five element teachers) satisfy the growing need for this kind of personal transmission of what I have learnt, then I hope these lessons will provide something which I cannot offer in any other way. The purist will complain that long-distance learning of this kind is not only far from ideal, but perhaps should not even be undertaken, because the student can be given so little feedback. But the purist is not confronted, as I am, with many hundreds of Chinese acupuncturists from all over their vast country longing to learn about five element acupuncture, and many more spread all over the world, eagerly learning whatever they can through my blogs.

CHAPTER 1

THE FIVE ELEMENTS

The guardian element

A study of the elements as abstract concepts is a study of the very essence of life itself. How, then, to find a way on to this vast landscape? Here nature comes to our aid, offering us evidence of the elements' manifestations in plant and tree, soil and pond. The changes wrought by the elements upon all things by the changing seasons can be seen, smelt, experienced within ourselves and thus provide the easiest first step towards developing our understanding. One advantage of studying nature in this way is that we do not at this early stage get caught up in all the awesomely complex layers which a human being adds to this picture. A rose is so simply and beautifully there, does not demand things of us, does not impinge upon us, does not, as far as we know, think the deep thoughts or have the deep feelings which make each of our lives so intricate and complicated. But, for all that, a rose, from seed, to bud, to withered petal, is as much a manifestation of the workings of each element in turn upon it as are its much more complex fellow manifestations in the human being, which create within each one of us those different aspects of our body and of the soul which animates this body.

Nature can therefore be used to help us more easily grasp the concepts of the different stages of this cycle as a first step along the path of our understanding. Thus to think of Wood as our body's spring or Metal as its autumn is to give us a first foothold on the complex human landscape. We then have to take the more difficult step of transferring such understanding to the processes of life within us. One way in is to look at how the elements unfold through the cycles of our life we know of as our ageing process. Here Wood can be seen as our childhood and youth, Fire early adulthood, Earth the time when we settle down to have our families, Metal the time of reflection in late maturity and Water the time when life is brought to a close before it restarts again in the shape of the next seed. Looking at the elements as parcels of our life in this way certainly helps us understand a little more about the differing qualities they impart to us, for we then learn that Earth always has about it some of the maturity we hope our thirties and forties bring us, Wood will retain into old age some of the freshness of our teens, and Metal, even in youth, will have some of the wisdom old age imparts.

We now need to extend our fledgling understanding of the elements by translating it on to the more complex human scale. And here we need to look at how the elements spread their spheres of influence over us through the medium of the organs of the body. We know that the ancient Chinese gave to each organ a function far exceeding those which Western medicine recognizes, endowing them with personal characteristics. We continue this tradition by calling each organ an official. Each is seen as fulfilling a function in the kingdom, much as officials would have surrounded the emperor in days long gone. Together they form a community, a kingdom of body and soul, in which each has specific responsibilities which contribute to the wellbeing of the whole.

We need to remember that the very structures over which the meridians pass, as well as the organs whose name they bear, are created by the energies of the elements flowing through these meridians. What we see as the superficial network of energy shown on the acupuncture chart interconnects below the surface with deeper pathways of energy emerging from the organs which give the meridians their names. We know that there are 12 meridians in all, and that each meridian relates to a specific organ or function, and that the 12 meridians thus formed relate to 12 different aspects of the elements' work. The meridians are the messengers which convey the organs' instructions to the remotest regions of this kingdom, and eventually to every cell in the body.

It is at the various sites at which the meridian network surfaces on the skin which we call acupuncture points that it becomes accessible to the interventions by the needle. Acupuncture points form entrances along the superficial meridian network to the structures lying hidden deep within us. These openings create tiny foci of energy at intervals along the meridians, and are the places at which energy can be drawn in, along and out of the meridians. Each is a powerful point of access to the energetic network which shapes us, body and soul. Each point reflects a different quality of energy, is regarded as having a unique function within the body of points and has been endowed since the earliest days with a unique name which reflects this function.

When viewed on the chart alone, the points may appear to lie at what could be considered random intervals along the meridians. And yet their positioning is far from arbitrary. They appear at sites where the energy feeding that particular part of the body encounters varying structures on its passage around the body, and are sited strategically along the meridian to encourage the smooth flow of that energy through and over these obstacles. Thus there are important points on all meridians as they encounter the obstacles created by the junction of joint to joint and tendon to tendon at important sites such as the knee, shoulder, vertebrae or neck. Points also provide interconnections with other meridians flowing through the same area, so that a particular function of one point drawing energy from one official is enhanced by a different form of energy drawn to it from another official crossing its path at that point. And yet so distinct are the individual functions of the points that one lying half an inch away from another on the same meridian is said to have a completely different action from that of its neighbour.

Most significantly of all, those areas of our body where we reach out to interact with the cosmos outside us, our hands to the air around us, our feet to the earth beneath us, are covered by the greatest concentration of important points, each finger and toe becoming a receptacle for the energies feeding the world, and in turn through these creating points of access to the outside world for the energies within us. These are the major sites of interaction between outside and inside, and places where this exchange of energy is most focused.

Each tiny acupuncture point will therefore be drawing to it energy brought to that unique site along a specific meridian. The acupuncturist's skill depends upon translating his/her understanding of these unique actions into a treatment protocol which is meaningful for that particular person on that particular day and at that particular stage of their life.

The energetic system formed initially of elements, subdivided first into officials, then into individual acupuncture points, reaches here an awesome degree of complexity comparable to that of Western medicine's multi-layered approach to the body. If we then interweave into every level of this complex structure that further layer of the soul within this body, we build up a symbolic representation of human beings in all our complexity.

THE GUARDIAN ELEMENT

At the heart of five element practice lies the understanding that each of us has a particular association with one element. This provides the focus for our life, endowing it with characteristics specific to that element. All the elements flow to a rhythm within us, their interplay determining who we are. Much as a painter can never put together an assembly of colours in exactly the same combination of pigments each time he mixes his paints, so the combination of elements which goes to make up our individual colour cannot be replicated elsewhere. Upon all of us they lay a hand of blessing, but one in particular has been selected as our special guardian to watch over and protect us, singling us out to bestow upon us the responsibility of our own individuality.

This element is known variously as the element of the causative factor of disease (CF) or the constitutional element. I call it our guardian element. I see it as protecting us as it guides us through life, being the place among the circle of elements where we can develop ourselves to our highest potential. The attributes this element imparts to us play an integral part in the way in which our energies become unbalanced, as well as in the way in which we grow and develop. Imbalance of any kind, whether of body or soul, is the result of some failure in the guardian element's ability to maintain balance.

In his book *In the Footsteps of the Yellow Emperor*, Peter Eckman (2007) gives an excellent overview of the various approaches to the constitutional element.* Of the concept of the CF he states: 'The technical definition of the CF is that it is the Element or Official whose chronic state of imbalance cannot be completely corrected by nature itself, and which in turn is responsible for producing or at least allowing imbalances to develop and persist in the other Elements or Officials. The CF thus becomes the primary focus for acupuncture treatment' (p.222). He adds: 'the various schools of Meridian Therapy in Japan and the Korean Constitutional style of acupuncture all specify a particular Element and Organ as the focus of treatment for each patient based on Five Element considerations, although they differ in regard to beliefs about when this predominant imbalance becomes established in life, and how invariant or changeable it may be over time' (pp.222–223).

There has thus always been much discussion as to whether we are born with this element as a dominant element, or whether it acquires its dominant position as a result of early trauma. Much of this discussion centres upon our differing beliefs as to whether we regard that element as being a site of weakness in the circle of the elements, or, by contrast, the focus for individual development, and thus potentially the site of our greatest strength.

If we view the constitutional element as revealing a weakness, treatment is seen as restoring that element to balance so that it can rejoin its fellow four in a dance of health. According to this perspective, this element's mark upon us, detected through sensory signals, is expected to fade and become neutral when good health is restored. If, however, we view this element as having a deeper function to perform, these diagnostic indicators are expected to lose their unbalanced expressions once treatment is focused upon this element (for example, the lack of red which the Fire element can show will change to a glowing pink), but will remain visible as the dominant expressions of the constitutional element even when it is in a state of health. Acupuncturists who base their practice upon the diagnosis and treatment of a constitutional element

---

* Eckman, P. (2007) *In the Footsteps of the Yellow Emperor*. San Francisco, CA: Long River Press.

(to be called from now on by the generic term of five element acupuncturists) must therefore decide which of these approaches they wish to adopt. The one I have come to accept is the second.

How we view our individual destinies hinges to a large extent upon the vision we each hold as to what life is about. I cannot accept that a human life can be nothing but the sum total of its inherited characteristics, determined purely by parental adequacies and inadequacies, with nothing added of some spark of individuality, giving to these characteristics something more and something different. It seems clear to me that the tiny soul, emerging untarnished from its mother's womb, brings with it into the world something uniquely its own, seen physically as its unique genetic imprint. Translated into the language of the elements, that imprint corresponds to a unique elemental imprint. I therefore see the guardian element as a blessing handed to us at our conception to provide a direction for our life, which is then shaped by the attributes and needs peculiar to this element.

Each of us in our uniqueness can thus be seen as reflecting reality from a slightly different angle. The tilt of that angle, its particular emphasis, is the product of the unique balance of the elements within us, and of the dominant position of one element. This forms the hub of the wheel of our life around which the other elements circle. It shapes our life for good, if we heed its warnings, or for ill, if we ignore them. All the other elements within us feel stronger if it is strong, grow weaker as it weakens. It is the focal point of each of our lives, dictating by its health or ill-health whether or not we will remain balanced within ourselves. It forms the core of our individuality. To those trained to detect the marks of the elements upon us, we appear each as a physical manifestation of the presence and power of this element within us.

We come into the world blessed with its special gift, and with this gift, the potential for using it either wisely or unwisely, of choosing to live within the shadows of its dark side rather than in its bright sunlight. And thus each of our five great guardians comes with its own dark companion, its Mephistopheles dogging its every footstep. Such positive, creative forces trail in their wake negative, destructive forces. Like everything else, an element can become a force for balance or imbalance. It can show us the way forward or bring us to a halt.

Our element imposes its own obligations upon us, for to live our life in balance requires us to live that life in tune with our element's demands. When we run true to its needs, we find a direction to our life which is fruitful. Many of my patients will tell me things like, 'I feel more myself now than I have ever felt', or, 'I know now who I am.' When we run counter to these needs, we lose our way, as though the undergrowth closes over the path we should take. Then our element turns from guardian into avenging angel, exacting revenge from us in the shape of ill-health and distress. To that extent we are not free, much as we are not free to choose when we are born, to which parents we are born, whether we are born poor or rich, tall or short, curly- or straight-haired.

In everything we do and everything we are we shout out our allegiance to this element. It puts its special seal upon us, and we bear its distinguishing mark printed upon us, no more to be altered than can the colour of our eyes or the size of our bones. We are who we are because we have received the gift of its patronage. So profound is the influence of this element, so all-pervasive is its mark upon us, that it lays a visible, palpable, audible signature upon us, writ large on our bodies, to be interpreted by eye and ear, and by touch and smell. It reveals itself by giving a specific colour to our face, a specific sound to our voice and a specific smell to our body.

My voice, for example, is not just a disembodied voice. It emerges from deep within me, and expresses who I am and what I am and how I am at any moment in time. It is the product of the unique interaction of the elements' work within me, and is sufficiently distinct that my voice-print can now open doors for me which will remain closed to any other voice. Similarly my smell and the colour upon my skin are unique to me and cannot be replicated elsewhere. They therefore offer unique diagnostic information if interpreted correctly.

Our element also endows us with a specific emotional orientation to our life which throws a patina of its own over all that we do. This emotional filter colours the way we see things, the way we respond to things, the way we move. It will affect the way we express ourselves in words as well as in action, and the way we perceive things. Our response to the stresses of life, as they act themselves out upon the elements, is therefore no haphazard process. The characteristics of our guardian element, determining as they do all that affects our life, will also determine the nature of our individual response to the difficulties we encounter. The way in which we fall ill will thus be as much influenced by our guardian element as will the way in which we fall in love, the jobs we do, the way we walk and talk and what we find funny or sad. Every facet of an individual life will be orientated towards that one segment of the complete cycle of the elements represented by this element.

The closest we come in the West to determining individual traits in a comparable way to this is when we categorize people as belonging to certain character types. The ancient medical concept of the humours, consigned long ago to gather dust on the shelves of medical libraries, also approaches this concept of the guardian element. Such systems of medicine, and others around the world, predominantly in the East, such as the Indian and Tibetan systems, all share a common belief that we shape our illnesses, that the type of person we are is a factor in the way in which we succumb to disease, and that we have a constitutional predisposition to certain imbalances.

The pursuit of the highest each one of us can achieve in a lifetime's efforts should be our life's aim. In acupuncture terms, it is acted out as the development of our guardian element to its highest potential. And this development is not a one-off thing, beginning at the start of treatment and coming to an end a few months later. It follows a continuous path throughout our life, as we develop and change, and the cycle of the elements turns again and again through each year and on to the next. Each time the cycle reaches the same point a year later it should do so at a higher level, representing another ring of experience added to our life, like the rings indicating a tree's age. And acupuncture treatment, experienced at the highest level, will accompany the patient on this journey through life, sometimes becoming more frequent as stresses occur and more support is needed, at other times infrequent, as the need for help recedes.

If we are to reach our true potential in body and soul, our guardian element must therefore be encouraged not only to reach a state of balance within itself but to stretch and challenge itself, and these two aims may sometimes clash. Our journey towards the fulfilment of our greatest potential may thus not always be a comfortable one as this element goads us towards change. Each treatment focused upon strengthening our guardian element can therefore be seen as a potential date with destiny.

CHAPTER 2

WOOD, FIRE, EARTH, METAL AND WATER

The five elements and their 12 officials
Introduction to the elements
The Wood element
The Fire element
The Earth element
The Metal element
The Water element
The qualities of the elements

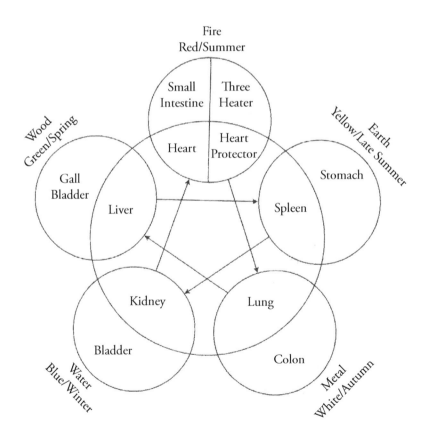

THE FIVE ELEMENTS AND THEIR 12 OFFICIALS

Five elements together create the circle of life. They are the elements Wood, Fire, Earth, Metal and Water. They delegate their work within us to 12 officials, each with a specific function. These are traditionally described as follows:

I	Heart	The supreme controller, the emperor of body, mind and spirit
II	Small Intestine	The official responsible for sorting the pure from the impure and transforming matter
III	Bladder	The controller of the storage of water
IV	Kidney	The controller of water
V	Heart Protector/ Circulation-Sex/ Pericardium	The official responsible for arterial and venous blood flow and for internal and external sexual secretions
VI	Three Heater/Triple Heater	The official responsible for the three burning spaces and for harmonizing the digestion of solid and liquid food
VII	Gall Bladder	The official in charge of decision-making
VIII	Liver	The official in charge of planning
IX	Lung	The receiver of qi energy from the heavens
X	Large Intestine/Colon	The official in charge of drainage and dregs
XI	Stomach	The official in charge of rotting and ripening food and drink
XII	Spleen	The minister of transport

Throughout this book I am retaining the use of Roman numerals for the officials, a convention in five element acupuncture, adding in brackets the more standard abbreviations to help readers who are unfamiliar with five element notation. There are two very important reasons for retaining this numbering system. It emphasizes the importance which five element acupuncture attaches to the Heart, the Supreme Controller. It is also a very useful reminder of the order of the officials along the Wei level of energy, as opposed to the Sheng cycle, and simplifies the diagnosis and annotation of Entry-Exit blocks (see Chapter 7).

Although Conception Vessel and Governor Vessel (Ren Mai and Du Mai) have also been given the numbers XIII and XIV respectively in the past, in practice these numerical abbreviations are now not often used, and have been replaced in five element terminology by the abbreviations CV and GV.

INTRODUCTION TO THE ELEMENTS

One of the difficulties I have in writing about the elements is that it is all too easy to fall into descriptions of stereotypes and all too difficult to attempt to describe how each of these precious qualities we regard as elements express themselves in the unique manifestation we recognize as a human being.

Over the years I have come to my own particular take on what I call an element type, only to find it constantly confounded by some expression of it in one of my patients which almost appears to contradict what I had perhaps too glibly assumed to be that element's characteristics. It is good to remind ourselves of the near-impossibility of type-casting ourselves in this way. As a five element acupuncturist who uses the elements as the tools of my trade, I would of course find it comforting if my patients appeared dressed in the primary colours they are given on my acupuncture chart, but that does not reflect the reality, which is that we all appear in a unique range of the most complex shadings. Here, then, I can only give expression to the elements in their simplest, most basic outlines, leaving it to each of us to round these out further from our own experience.

Before I start, though, I have to pause, for I find it easier to write about some elements than others, and have had to think deeply why this should be so. I must present my apologies to the first two elements, Wood and Fire, each for a different reason. Once I move on to Earth I start to feel myself relax, and with Metal and Water I plunge with relief into the deeper and more rarefied areas of life which are the regions I find it easiest to write about.

What is it then that blocks my thoughts when I think of the Wood element? It may have something to do with its sheer simplicity and directness. It is just there, standing foursquare in front of me. It hinders my vision beyond and to the side of it, demanding attention. It has no use of subtleties or nuances. It says outright what it thinks and its thoughts are clear and single-tracked, expressing in no uncertain terms a view of life which welcomes certainty.

Perhaps its very straightforwardness is a challenge to me, for I have to meet it head on and the words I find myself using to describe it are down-to-earth, simple and forceful, and require little of the subtlety and poetry I enjoy with other elements.

As I write, I find myself wanting to veer away from what I see as the knock-for-knock encounter Wood demands of me, a meeting of myself with some force which pushes at me. My words frequently take on a critical tinge as though the qualities of Wood I am trying to describe arouse resistance in me and show their negative sides. Perhaps I envy such a forthright approach to life, one that I may wish to emulate but cannot, and this envy reveals itself in some negative colouring. How easy it must be, I think, to see life in such simple outlines, to want things so clearly and to express my dissatisfactions so forcefully if I don't get what I want. To these, though, I must also add some personal experiences of the Wood element in my close family which have shaped my understanding, sometimes positively, sometimes negatively. So I cannot approach Wood neutrally. It always evokes some stirrings of disturbance within me, much like those I experience as winter starts giving way to spring and change is in the air, making me restless.

These confessions made, (and Wood, I feel, will accept them in the forthright spirit which is one of its hallmarks), I can now move on to its territory within the five element circle, opening the gate a little to let in a breath of fresh spring air, a welcome draught of new life and optimism with which it is good to start this brief journey round the elements.

THE WOOD ELEMENT: The guardian element of hope and renewal
Picture the immense flatness of a winter landscape. Nothing stirs. All is lifeless. No flicker of movement for the eye to behold. Even the air seems hushed into silence, a dead and heavy weight, through which any sound that comes to us resonates as though in some high vaulted chapel. Nature cowers down, hiding from the cold. And yet as the days slowly lengthen something starts to stir, like some slight itch upon the surface of things. A ripple seems to flow over the land as tiny eruptions break through earth and bough, first appearing as no more than slight bumps along the surface of things, then, as they grow bolder and the air into which they push grows milder, they announce themselves as shadings of green, always green, as nature unravels itself and announces new life in the shape of a bud.

We have to marvel at the power of it, the sheer guts required to gather together all that is necessary to break through frozen earth and lifeless branch, drawing out into the daylight a myriad of tiny celebrations of the renewal of life. There is something bloody-minded about such audacity. To bring life where life appeared extinguished requires a form of stubbornness which is the hallmark of that force of life we call the element Wood. Strength is required to focus sufficient energy upon a single point to draw out into the daylight the seed lying dormant deep within, and then to move to the next spot and do the same again and again, until the whole landscape gleams with a vibrant shimmer of renewed life.

Wood is our structuring force, shaping our future for us, and by each of its actions defining a tiny segment of that future. The doing of things is its territory, and these things must be done according to the plans it has decreed for them. It places a blueprint upon life, each bud bearing within it its own little plan for the future growth of mature plant, tree or human being.

The world presents itself to Wood as a place of infinite potential, of things waiting to be done, so many, indeed, that it is always somewhat impatient to get on with them lest something slips past. It has such a zest for all the activities life presents us with, such sheer enjoyment in the doing of things and in the challenges such actions possess, that this enthusiasm gives a quality of youthful optimism to all it does. It is the most uninhibited of all elements, announcing its presence with all the vigour with which spring bursts out of winter. In its eyes, life always wears its brightest spring colours, and at some level, however balanced it is, it always harbours some slight resentment at being asked to put away childish things and accept in their place the more sober life maturity demands of us.

Wood likes to stride forward on the field of action, which is where it feels most at home, and any restriction to its freedom of movement will be countered by an expression of its emotion which we call anger. We use this word in the sense of a natural forcefulness, a desire to get on with things. This emotion can turn into frustration when its natural vigour is baulked in any way, as it responds to the suppression of its energy with the anger of a child forced to sit at home, whilst the sun and its fellows call it out to play.

Wood spreads the pale green colours of spring-time over our face, and its smell is that of fresh vegetation. Its voice reveals its need for control. We call it a shouting voice, and buried within it there is always something of the clipped sound of someone wanting to be in command. And these commands are carried out by its two officials, the Liver and Gall Bladder, the one involved in the planning of things, the other in the decisions necessary to carry out these plans.

Patient profile
A Wood patient of mine, now aged 45, has been coming for treatment for the past eight years, and I now see him about twice or three times a year. He

suffered originally from constant digestive troubles and headaches, which had started in his twenties. I traced some of the cause of this back to a difficult time he had had at university where he had felt himself hemmed in by the course of studies he had chosen, a sign of Wood's dislike of being in a situation it cannot control. He was initially impatient at how slowly things appeared to be improving, and nearly stopped treatment early on until I explained quite firmly the need to give it time to work. Here I found myself taking over control and providing the firm structure within which Wood feels at home.

He is a delightful patient, coming willingly now for treatment whenever he needs to, doing all I suggest to ensure that his lifestyle contributes to his health, and full of the bounce which is so characteristic of Wood. This can be the easiest element to treat if we get our approach to our patient right and stay firmly in control of treatment, because all it wants is to feel better in order to get back out there and get on with things again. The soft comforts of the treatment room, with their invitation to relax and let go, are not where Wood feels most at home. It would far rather be out there initiating things, doing things, getting on with things, looking here and there to see what needs to be done, each little action it undertakes another bud bursting into life.

THE FIRE ELEMENT: The guardian element of relationship
Wood, the child amongst the elements, hands us over to Fire, to the time of the young adult. The single bud, once so preoccupied with its own renewal, becomes aware of the other buds upon the bough. With Fire we enter the world of relationships.

Here I have to declare another interest, for this is my particular territory, the segment of the five element circle which is my home. Nothing is more difficult than to write about what is closest to oneself, and to ask that I write about the Fire element is no exception. It stirs emotions within me that I try to hide within what I am writing, but colour it nonetheless, so that my words often come out as slightly stilted, as though my mind is setting them down, but my heart, so central to the Fire element, is not in them. I have tried many times to start these few words afresh, and always return with something a little different but still lacking some quality of truthfulness which I feel I give to the other elements.

One of the difficulties I have is in describing the sheer complexity of the Fire element, which has two very distinct aspects, reflecting its four officials. One side I call Inner Fire, the other Outer Fire, and they have very different qualities. It is almost as though we are given two Fire guardian elements to work with. With Inner Fire I am in a literal sense at home. Outer Fire is less familiar territory to me, and yet shares enough with me to be a little confusing and awaken some feelings of disturbance for its very familiarity. Luckily, too, in my difficulty I am helped by Fire's sheer accessibility and openness. Like Wood, it is there in front of me, the most yang of all the elements, its arms flung wide to the world as nature bursts into blossom in summer, revealing the very innermost workings of each of spring's tightly clasped buds. All is now open to the gaze. Fire's blossoms embrace to the full the warmth of high summer, opening themselves eagerly to the world. This openness to the world around it can expose it to attack, and it must learn to develop the protective mechanisms we all need if we are to live productively in a world crowded with other people, each potentially an area of conflict and confusion which it is the Fire element's task to resolve.

And this complex grouping of officials within the one element, the only one to shelter four partners, indicates how vital to the functioning of the whole this element is. As the Heart at its very core continuously pumps the life-blood for body and soul, it lies encircled within the arms of Fire's two all-encompassing officials, the Three Heater and the Heart Protector. The Three Heater is perhaps the most complex of all officials, so diffuse and widespread is its task to harmonize all the disparate, sometimes conflicting needs of the other officials. The Heart Protector, in charge of the extensive, far-flung network of blood vessels, roams widely, and, like the Three Heater, is unhampered by that attachment to locality which an association with an organ lends to all the other officials. These two Outer Fire officials act as roving ambassadors for the Heart, as well as forming the Heart's bodyguards, often working unnoticed to bring order to the kingdom to allow the Heart to do its work of ruling with justice and fairness.

We then move closer to the Heart, and to an organ, the Small Intestine, which in the family of officials is tucked closest to the Heart, its yang to the Heart's yin. We can gain some understanding of the importance of this official if we look at its superficial pathway as it runs up over the arm to criss-cross the shoulders before marching beside the Bladder and Governor Vessels up to the neck and head. Only these three officials can be seen as supporting the most densely weight-bearing aspect of the back between them, providing the very backbone of our energy. Here we can see illustrated the Small Intestine's importance to the Fire element, giving it, and the Heart within it, that deep strength to survive come what may. Some of the playful joy which summer brings is here tempered with the need to ensure that nothing threatens the Heart. This makes it a tough official, burdened with getting things right with each beat of the Heart. All this crucial work demands that it must be endlessly watchful, aware of what is going on around, with a speed of thought and action enabling quick decisions to be made, obstructions to be removed and problems to be ironed out promptly.

And then to the very core of us, to the Heart, the Supreme Controller, the Lord and Emperor of the kingdom of body and soul, the very essence of our being. How fortunate he is to be surrounded by such a dedicated team of defenders, there to fulfil his every whim, to run and carry, to harry the other officials to do their work, whilst he sits on his throne directing all, the Small Intestine at his feet busily sifting and sorting, sifting and sorting. When both are working efficiently, each heartbeat proceeds calmly, unnoticed by us when we are healthy. But should even the slightest hitch occur in the smooth workings of this powerhouse, we become instantly aware of intimations of chaos, as if danger threatens every part of us. Even one missed heartbeat, one erratic pounding of this usually so steady organ, and the kingdom starts to tremble.

The Small Intestine's work in maintaining the Heart's power is evidence of the ability of both officials to keep going come what may. The Heart only gives up at death, its yang companion matching it beat for beat until that last moment. These two officials therefore always have something about them of the seriousness of those confronted with what is life-threatening, a patina of gravity tingeing all that they do. Sometimes it is difficult to recognize in them the characteristics commonly associated with the Fire element, those of joyousness and laughter, for they only show these clearly when their work is done to their satisfaction and they have accomplished all that needs to be done, rare moments of repose between bouts of intense activity.

In the two Outer Fire officials we see Fire's face turned more easily towards the brightness of summer, its season, with all its lightness and joy. There is an openness to this aspect which Inner Fire may aspire to but rarely achieves. The Outer Fire officials guard the Heart in their own way, but have no need of such earnest unremitting work. Provided their defences are strong, they have time to play and enjoy themselves on the battlements, showing in balance that glow of joy which spreads happiness to those around them like a sun warming all with its rays. For Fire's emotion is joy and its sound is laughing, its colour red and its smell scorched.

When Fire loses its balance, the imbalances within Inner and Outer Fire differ. Inner Fire will show an increased level of activity, a kind of hyperactivity, which may be reflected physically in an increase in heart rate. It will resort to a confused state of constant self-questioning and doubt, misjudging what it needs to do to keep the whole mechanism of body and soul together. Eager to do something, it may become too frenzied, too preoccupied with getting everything right, often confusing others with the signals it sends out, above all through its speech, which is one of the main channels through which the Small Intestine sends out the Heart's instructions. Hesitant or garbled thoughts and speech may be a sign of disturbance in Inner Fire as confused messages are sent to and fro in an attempt to keep the kingdom under control.

Outer Fire will show a different kind of imbalance. It forms the outer ramparts of Fire's defences, standing beyond the inner sanctum of the Heart. If not sufficiently fortified, such defences are susceptible to attack from without, bringing in their wake signs of the vulnerability characteristic of this aspect of Fire. It is the line of Fire which faces the world directly, the first place of interaction between us and the world around us. If it is damaged in any way, it will be vulnerable to approaches made by others, retreating behind a shell of often self-inflicted pain. Unsure how to respond, it may shrink back within itself if it feels unable to cope, becoming a shadow of that bright and open Fire aspect we associate with Outer Fire in balance.

Treatment for both follows the same pattern to start with, at least four treatments being addressed at the Outer Fire officials. Thereafter their paths will diverge if we decide to move on to treat Inner Fire. The purpose behind this is to ensure that Fire's outer protective wall is sufficiently strengthened at the start, whatever aspect of Fire we diagnose. Since it is often difficult to distinguish between the two sides of Fire, these first few treatments also provide an opportunity to see how far the Three Heater and Heart Protector accept this treatment. If they respond well, we will remain on the periphery and continue to treat Outer Fire, but if we find that we are not addressing the right aspect of Fire, the Inner Fire officials will start to show their dissatisfaction as their needs continue to be ignored. We then move inwards to treat the Heart and Small Intestine.

Patient profile

The examples of the two aspects of Fire I give below show these different characteristics clearly, and will help illustrate what is often a difficult distinction to make, for, whatever their differences, both aspects reside within the Fire element and have many features in common. For Inner Fire I have chosen a patient who came to me for help with feelings of despair. She was in what she described as an unsatisfactory marriage, tolerated for her children's sake, and could see no future for herself wherever she looked. What was obvious from the initial diagnosis was how hard she was working at trying to sort her problems out herself. In some ways I could sense that she felt she was somehow failing herself by asking for help from me. She listened carefully to what I said, but needed to make her thoughts her own, clearly thinking things over in front of me and then agreeing or disagreeing with me. There was something here of what we will see is Earth's capacity to process things, yet the difference lies in the speed at which that processing is done and the ability to hear and to process at the same time. We will find that Earth likes to take in one thought at a time so that it can work through each thoroughly. The Small Intestine, on the other hand, can and has to take in many things at the same time, thoughts, words and actions, and will attempt to make sense of all of them as quickly as it can to help the Heart maintain balance. How successfully it does this will depend on its level of balance.

In imbalance, it may jumble all these together, confusing both itself and others. My patient gave many examples of such confusion, and her somewhat erratic behaviour, obviously difficult for her partner to cope with, turned out to be one of the major areas of disturbance in their relationship. Treatment to help the Inner Fire officials deal more smoothly with all the often conflicting demands placed upon them helped steady her so that the image she now conveys to others is no longer so confusing. In turn, this newly found balance led her to sort out her marital problems in a more constructive way. We could say that her Heart regained control of its own power, and was able to lead her in a stable direction.

Outer Fire imbalances appear as a breakdown of Fire's defensive mechanism, and such people show a high level of concern about how to deal with people around them. This may lead to their shrinking away from contact with other people because of an inability to protect themselves, in this way refusing to engage with others because of the possibility of hurt against which they have less and less protection. They may also misjudge the nature of their contacts, opening up to some people unwisely and fending off others unnecessarily. Although apparently on the outer periphery of Fire, there is what can be regarded as a predominantly yin quality to this aspect of Fire conveyed by its yin aspect, the Heart Protector function, whereas Inner Fire always has about it some of the yang strength of the Small Intestine, standing as close sentinel to the yin Heart official.

An example of Outer Fire is provided by another of my patients. With him I can already feel myself relaxing and smiling, sinking back almost with relief as I move from Inner to Outer Fire. From the start he was very eager to grasp the opportunity to change and develop which his treatment brought him. He just wants people around him to be happy, and then he is happy, and this includes me as his practitioner. He is always delighted when he is able to tell me how good he is feeling and how much his life is changing for the better.

When he first came, he had a kind of passivity about himself, almost as though he had made a deal with himself to accept life as it was, however inadequate and unhappy he felt, and had decided not to put too many demands upon its ability to give him happiness. He said that his relationship with his partner was good, and yet he spoke without any of the joy the Heart gives when it is truly engaged, and I could see that there were deep issues between them on which he was taking a passive role, almost abdicating his right to assert himself. The feeling of resignation was very strong.

Treatment directed at strengthening the outer defences of the Heart gave him the courage to stand up a little, both at home and at work. He became much more obviously joyful, able to approach a mother he had last seen some years back and reconcile himself to a sister with whom he had had a difficult relationship since childhood. His judgements about his relationships to other people became more appropriate, and he was able to keep his defences up against those which might be harmful, something he had so obviously failed to do in the past.

As both of my two Fire patients moved towards greater balance, the sensory signals of distress in their element changed, so that their colour took on a healthier pink glow, their smell became less strongly scorched and laughter was at last heard to return to their voices. The joy lurking always beneath the surface ready to break out was more openly expressed by Outer Fire, but my Inner Fire patient, too, revealed a greater capacity to show warmth. And yet she retains always some quality which reflects Inner Fire's deep responsibilities, a kind of serious joyfulness, and will rarely show the overt expressions of joy which my other patient now feels more able to offer those around him.

THE EARTH ELEMENT: The guardian element of home and hearth
Wood and Fire, the elements of spring and summer, direct their energies away from themselves. They are both instigators of action, moving out towards the world. Both, in their differing ways, give. But as the summer draws to a close, nature sinks back into itself. The movement outwards of spring and summer gives way to a movement inwards as the year withdraws into itself and tilts towards the dark. The elements turn their energies slowly inwards and start, instead, to receive. Earth lies at this turning-point of the year, when our energies begin to coil in upon themselves after the intense activities of spring and summer. Earth gathers to itself the harvest of Wood's actions and Fire's relationships and turns them into the nourishment which feeds all life. It is

Mother Earth in all her abundance, the womb of life, bringing forth all that nourishes us. Like the ground beneath our feet upon which all rests, Earth is the foundation which supports us. It is the hub of the wheel of the elements, a pivot around which the other elements turn.

It represents, too, the physical mother who bears us, and will show by its balance or imbalance the nature of our relationship with our mother, just as Metal will show the nature of our relationship with our father. The movement outwards towards the beloved which is Fire's expression of love becomes, in Earth, a movement inwards, a drawing towards itself of the beloved, both to nourish and to be nourished.

Like Fire, Earth is concerned with people, for it is there to nourish them, but where Fire relates like a lover stretching out to his beloved, Earth relates like a mother drawing her child to her breast. And since it needs to receive before it can give out, it must itself be fed before it can feed others. It therefore has a dual role, alternating between the hungry child demanding food and the satisfied mother ready to nourish others. Earth is always involved in this two-way process. It draws nourishment from outside, both physically in the form of food to our mouth, and mentally and spiritually in the form of thoughts and feelings, and all this it processes and passes on to the other elements. It acts as a channel from outside to inside, and is always either emptying itself or filling itself. In that sense, since everything it takes in has to be passed immediately on, it can be regarded as constantly empty and hungry, never replete. There is thus a necessary neediness about the Earth element, for it knows that it must nourish itself before satisfying the demands the other elements make upon it.

So relentless is our need for nourishment that Earth can itself feel drained and empty. And thus where Fire in its imbalance will ache with the pain of its Heart's wounding, Earth can ache with the pain of hunger, and, like some parched and arid desert, can give nothing of itself when it has nothing left to give. Fire will always wish to give something, until its embers fade and die, for that very act of giving feeds it, kindling its flames to renewed life. Earth, denied its own nourishment, must hold to itself all that it can bestow, else it will starve, and if it is troubled, it has to become selfish. Taking what it should be giving, it stands hungry before its own empty larder, demanding of others that they replenish it. For deep within Earth lies the ghost of a starving child.

Earth's two officials are the Stomach, which processes the food we eat, and at a deeper level also processes our thoughts and feelings, and the Spleen which is the servant of our energy, the body's distributor, there to fetch and carry whatever the other elements need. It is a vehicle for the use of others, a constant conveyor belt, distributing Earth's nourishment throughout the regions of our body and soul.

Earth appears on our faces as a pale yellow colour, in our voices as a lilting tone, like a mother singing a lullaby, and upon our bodies as a sweet smell. Its dominant emotion is understanding and empathy with all that it draws to itself. It has the capacity to feel with us, sympathy in its original sense of the word. In balance, it will have that deep feeling for others' pain of a mother experiencing all her child's sorrows and joys.

Patient profile

An Earth patient came with badly swollen ankles and stomach cramps. These symptoms had started shortly after he had been promoted at work and moved to an office of his own. What Earth craves above all is the company of others. It needs to be in the centre of things, not on the periphery, as this patient felt he had become as a result of his promotion. He now dreaded going to his lonely office each day, having become too isolated from the rest of the group to function properly.

The Earth element was showing its distress in different ways. It could not digest food properly, leading to stomach cramps, and it could not distribute properly, causing the fluid to accumulate around his ankles. Treatment of the Earth element increased the amount of energy supplying the Earth officials, and, as they gradually returned to balance, his swollen ankles and stomach disorders improved. As part of his treatment, I encouraged him to move other people back into his office, and this he then did. He told me that he felt much easier in himself now that he was no longer alone, and the standard of his work had improved. He realized that he had been using numerous pretexts to leave his room before, simply to be with other people. Now he felt once more at the heart of things, surrounded by a support group, that home for which all Earth people yearn.

THE METAL ELEMENT: The guardian element of purity

All the good nourishment Earth has produced is harvested for storage in our granaries at the end of the summer, and the year turns into autumn, the season of the element Metal. Metal stands at the end of the cycle of activity started by Wood, just as autumn brings spring's work to a close. Autumn is a season of loss, a time of regret when we pause and take stock as we mourn the passing of the year. The trees, stripped of their leaves, reveal themselves in all their stark outlines, like flesh stripped from the bone revealing the skeleton beneath. This is a time when we see things for what they are.

Here, in this segment of the five element circle, I feel the most naturally at ease, for some reason I have still to fathom clearly, for I seem to appreciate and understand the subtle depth of Metal's qualities as though they reflect the ability to achieve something I always strive for. One explanation for this may lie in the fact that of the many people who have helped me deeply in my life the majority have been Metal, and I still call upon their deep wisdom.

Where Earth, the nurturing element, is the element of the mother, Metal is that of the father, both the father who bears us, and that transcendental manifestation of all that lies beyond and above our everyday life, the spiritual presence represented by 'our Father that art in Heaven'. Our image of Earth is that of our feet firmly attached by gravity to the ground. That of Metal is of our arms outstretched towards the heavens above.

Metal rules over the widest domain of all the elements, extending from the Lungs as our organ of intake to the Large Intestine, our principal organ of excretion. It connects us through our breath to the vast breath of the universe rhythmically breathing in and out beyond us. And this awareness of all that lies beyond itself draws Metal's attention away from the small considerations of our everyday life up towards those things which soar eternally beyond life and death. Metal forms our bridge to the great worlds beyond. And its task is to translate all that happens within the tiny, apparently insignificant span of each of our lives into something of meaning within the greater context of all that exists.

Metal waits until all the bustle of spring and summer is past before setting to work to pare away all that is insignificant, retaining only that which it considers worth keeping if the future is to gain any value from its past. If life is to be worth anything, it is Metal that assesses what that worth could be. Where Fire weighs all things upon the scales of love, Metal weighs them upon the scales of their value. Its task is to ensure that the great cycle of activity starting with Wood does not fade away into insignificance.

Metal represents not only the air we breathe, but also that essence which nature passes on to feed the renewal of life each year. Not all withers away to nothing in autumn. The dead leaves, broken down by the forces of rain and wind, release into the ground trace elements which nourish the ground in which the future seed will grow. The quality of what has been deposited in the soil in autumn will determine the strength of next year's growth. Without air, nothing can live, and without trace elements the soil cannot nurture the rebirth of life. Without Metal's quality, the work of all the other elements would be as nothing, valueless.

So strong is Metal's determination to deal only with what is valuable and pure, that it will set itself and others the highest standards, often finding it difficult itself to live up to them. Metal people are perfectionists, being unable to finish a thing until it is exactly as they want it. They have difficulty in accepting that they have done the best they can, because that best is never enough. And having always some lingering suspicion that they could have done better, they can be reluctant to let things go.

Balanced Metal will encourage the Large Intestine to remove what is no longer useful. But when it is out of balance it will lose its ability to distinguish between what should be retained and what should be discarded, and then it will function uneasily, at times holding on to everything, at others letting everything go. And this is how we can become constipated or have loose bowels. Such imbalances will also block us at other levels, as Metal's inability to discard what is no longer of value to us mentally or spiritually causes our minds and spirits to become sluggish.

If Metal people have not eliminated what is valueless to them, they may feel unclean inside, and overcompensate either by becoming excessively scrupulous about their appearance, always being immaculately groomed in public, or by appearing unwashed and unkempt. Both are different reflections of a sense of inner worthlessness and loss of self-respect.

In their search for what lies beyond themselves, Metal people always feel there is something out there which they must strive to reach. In balance, they will experience this as something further on, beyond them, a goal to be achieved. Out of balance, they will experience this as something further back which has eluded them, an opportunity missed, a cause for regret. Metal is the element that most sighs for what might have been and now can never be. Once its energy becomes unbalanced, this sense of past failure can become so crippling that a person lives only in the past, looking back with longing eyes to a time when things might have been different. And this yearning for some past time which never was can cut Metal people off from the present, making them feel as though they are no longer connected to things. Life can then seem empty and meaningless, its purpose no longer clear.

And there is a sadness deep within Metal, for this seeker after the perfect knows that, search as it will, it can never find the perfect thing for which it is looking. It weeps for all our imperfections. It weeps because it knows that at the heart of Wood's bud of hope lies nestling death, life's eternal shadow. Thus grief is Metal's emotion. Its colour is white, the colour of the shroud, its smell is that of autumn leaves trodden underfoot, and its voice mourns for the passing of all things.

Where Earth people may feel that their mother has not nurtured them, Metal people may experience a feeling of loss in relation to their father, as though he has cut himself off from them. And they will feel deep within themselves that they must somehow re-establish this lost connection. We seek comfort from our mother and respect from our father, and if a father is unable to enter into a close relationship with his child, that child will experience this rejection as an attack upon its own sense of self-value. Metal people feel diminished in their own eyes if other people do not give them the respect they crave. Since they judge all things by their value, they will judge other people's feelings towards them in terms of how much these people value them. This differs from Fire, which will judge other people's feelings in terms of the love they are allowed to offer them.

Patient profile

A young Metal patient came for treatment after breaking down whilst at university. He had great difficulty in studying, and was not sure whether the course he had chosen was what he really wanted to do. He came from a family of high achievers, and had a great deal of pressure placed upon him to succeed academically. He felt that he was a failure in their eyes, believing that nothing he could do would ever match their achievements. There was a feeling of pointlessness to everything he did, that emptiness which makes itself felt in Metal people when they feel that they lack others' respect. Living in the shadow of such a dominant, successful family, he had never been able to establish a true sense of his own identity. It was little wonder that he felt, as he said, as though he could be 'blown away in a puff of smoke'. He had lost contact with his very essence, that quality which Metal imparts to all that we do.

He was having difficulty in functioning properly in the atmosphere of self-doubt and failure which increasingly oppressed him. In effect, he was being stifled by life. His breakdown was the final stage in this history of personal misery. He could no longer see any worth in what he was doing. Already feeling cut off from life by a growing sense of failure, he felt there was no point in continuing.

Treatment was directed at strengthening the Metal element. As its energy improved, he regained a sense of connectedness with things. This helped reinforce the feeling that there was some point to his life. With a greater sense of self-worth, he began to re-assess his relationship with his family, seeing them now more as relationships of equals in which he, too, had something of value to offer. As he learnt to assess the value of his own life in true terms, he was able to discard what was valueless to him, including his own idea of himself as a failure. After a few months of treatment, he felt strong enough to return to university, but decided to change the subject he wanted to study. This decision reflected his newly acquired conviction that it was he, not his father, who must be the only judge of what was right for himself.

THE WATER ELEMENT: The medium of life
The cycle of life gives a further twist to the wheel of the elements, an endless channel through which life passes on its way towards eternity, each element a prayer-bead slipping slowly through the hands of time. And the thread along which these beads are strung is held softly, but tenaciously, in the flowing hands of the last and most mysterious of elements, Water, with which everything comes full circle. For Water is the great unifier, drawing all things, not to a close, but to a closed circle, in its great strength refusing to allow even mountain-ranges to stand in the way of its quest for unity, and slicing relentlessly but gently drop by drop both through hard rock-face and soft sand, until it finds its way back to itself.

The great wheel of the elements, endlessly turning, rests in turn upon one of its five spokes, each a moment in the cycle from birth to death and on to birth again. And each turn of the wheel echoes the rise and fall of life, the moment of birth finding the little bud of Wood peering hopefully out of the dead land into the new world of spring, before calling upon Fire's warmth to ripen it to maturity. And on the wheel turns, bearing with it the fruit of Fire's labours to drop into Earth's ample lap as food to sustain life, where Metal, watching from afar, swoops down to extract one pure and precious jewel worthy of bearing on high.

The moment at which Metal soars upwards to the skies above is the point of our greatest detachment from the whole, the peak of our individuality. And as the wheel turns gently on to float in Water, Metal's great yearning to find its lost paradise is effortlessly answered, for Water bears within it that knowledge of paradise regained so desperately and vainly sought by Metal. We have reached the moment in the cycle where we merge ourselves in the whole again, drawn down into the watery depths of all that is. As the waters reclaim us we yield ourselves to them, under the pressure of their gentle but relentless force abandoning all attempts at soaring up.

In Water there echoes the profound and age-old memory of a time when all things were one, before the universe burst outwards into existence, flinging matter far out into the furthest reaches of space. It was Water's eternal flow and rhythm which gradually shaped the world, existing as it did before Earth was born, before sun, moon and stars lit up the skies and warmed the seed of

Man sufficiently to coax him into existence inside that very microcosm of the original unity of the universe, the watery bed of his first cell.

Down from the outermost reaches of space Water has floated, combining, condensing and endlessly changing shape and form before spreading itself in a film upon the face of the earth to become the seed-bed of all life. For what great purpose we may only dimly perceive, it prepares the land to receive the great gift of life, for it is the medium through which everything passes on its way to becoming alive.

Wherever it encounters obstacles to its own smooth ebb and flow, there it must set to work, indifferent to all but its own absorbing need to envelop and smooth away whatever it finds deflecting its unifying tide. All it wants is to be left in peace to be itself, floating at one with its fellows in the billowing ocean of all that is, and for this right it will work hard and long, silently but inexorably fighting its eternal battle to force into defeat whatever gets in its way. A master of disguises, it has learnt to don a multiplicity of masks, evading capture by transforming itself. Fleeing alike the summer's heat and winter's freezing breath, it will abruptly change its watery home to live elusively amongst misty vapours or defended by barriers of solid ice whenever it feels threatened by extinction, biding its time and awaiting the moment when it can return to its watery shape once more. Like some eternal cuckoo, it will make its home wherever it finds itself, gracefully taking up new residence amongst both icy wastes and misty clouds.

Apparently passive and lazy, it offers no resistance to the endless buffetings of wind and cold and heat, emerging victorious where less flexible elements would long since have succumbed, its very passivity proving its strength. By itself each of those tiny and insignificant drops together forming the great oceans of the sea and the billowing clouds of the air is too weak to survive such onslaughts, but banded together with its fellows it becomes a terrifying opponent against which all the might of the other elements is as nothing. If allowed the freedom to flow as it wishes, Water will become life's soothing and merciful companion, bringing harmony and wholeness to all it touches. All life is awash with its energy as it flows through our veins and nourishes our cells, but under threat this life-giving force can overwhelm and destroy, consigning Wood's hopeful buds to a soggy death, extinguishing Fire, flattening the Earth and drowning Metal's precious gifts fathoms deep.

A raging torrent one moment, a stagnant puddle the next, held tight in a glacier's icy grasp, or floating softly down in the morning dew, it has the power to be all things to all men, but in so being fears that it may be nothing in particular to itself. Its very changeability safeguards it from destruction, endowing it with the special gift of endless transformation, and yet its own unpredictability frightens it, for it is never sure where it is at any moment, for the next may well find it elsewhere. This bestows upon it both the comforting gift of survival and the terror of knowing that but one brief moment's isolation from its companions is sufficient to render it powerless, an insignificant raindrop abandoned on a leaf to be brushed away indifferently by the merest breath of wind or evaporated by the first rays of the morning sun.

Winter is Water's season. All things cower down to survive its bitter cold, huddling together, like those droplets in the ocean, to find protection in bulk against the harsh conditions outside. The land opens its arms and pulls inside it all it can lay hold upon, the trees and bushes, cleared of unnecessary leaves, sinking lower and sending all their vitality and strength deep into their roots to guard against extinction. Winter is the time when nature has to trust the most to its own powers of regeneration, requiring of us the greatest courage. As the cold, harsh days pass slowly by, we cannot know whether we have amassed sufficient strength to survive until spring. Now we will discover whether the year's busy work in gathering together its reserves has been sufficient, before winter's cold curtain descends upon the land.

Water shapes us, as it shapes all things. It is the flow and rhythm of life's sap within us. With the structure and definition the other elements provide, it is channelled into the narrow confines of our cells, the delicate arteries of our blood and the myriad pathways of fluid which feed our hormones and our tears. And the Kidney and the Bladder are the officials over which Water has control.

Water is our will to survive. All Water people will be endowed with some of its implacable strength. Despite apparently bending to the whim of those who press against them, it is they who finally prevail, echoing in their strength the inexorable progress of flood water as it drowns the land. And yet, strong and brave as this element is, buried far beneath its flowing surface there lies within it an echo of that terror of the deep which we all feel. There is in Water some of the fear nature must feel as winter covers the land, an ever-present anxiety underlying all that Water does, and fear is its emotion. That which is risky is its familiar territory. In balance, Water's fear is a protective barrier which enables it to survive, acting as a warning to move away from situations which are too dangerous. When it is out of balance, it may become confused, and engage in activities it should be counselling itself against.

Its colour is the blue of the ocean, it has the sharp smell of stagnant water, and the sound of its voice can be the hesitant gurgle of a stream finding its way gently between the rocks of a river bed, or the monotonous and far-distant murmur of the sea.

Water people embody the mysterious qualities we associate with their physical counterpart in nature. They are elusive, unwilling to be pinned down, often fickle in their need to escape situations which prove too rigid for them. And yet, unlike Metal, they are not loners, being seldom content with their own company, for they have a greater need even than that of Earth to feel secure, seeking situations and company which reassure them that they are safe. And their fear will drive them to move away to safer pastures elsewhere as soon as they start to feel threatened.

Where Earth needs the company of others like a hub of a wheel needs its spokes, Water needs their company as a grain of sand buried among a million others, desiring above all to be at one with all that is around it. Water people will try to fit into any situation, eager to adapt to the company they find themselves in. In their flexibility, they can change their mind to suit what is wanted of them, appearing to others as inconsistent, and yet to themselves this ability to change course and opinion at will is reassuring confirmation of their own capacity to survive.

The lives of Water people will show an almost inexorable progress towards some goal. They may appear to be vacillating, moving to and fro, unsure of what they should do, and yet, like the turbulent waves of the ocean hiding the deep and steady pull of the current beneath, at some profound level inside themselves they know where they are going. They are ambitious, and will not stop until they have achieved what they have set out to do. The sense of potential failure haunting each Metal person is alien to Water, which cannot contemplate the possibility of failing to fulfil whatever ambition it has.

Patient profile

A Water patient came for treatment suffering from anxiety attacks and severe back pain as a result of an accident during a parachute jump for charity. He had only been given the sketchiest training before making the jump, but his unbalanced Water energy had led him to accept a challenge someone else might well have refused. In its imbalance, his Water energy had lost the ability to protect him from danger, leading him instead straight towards it. In effect, he engineered himself into a situation which finally magnified his own fear.

There had been numerous incidents in his life to suggest that his Water energy had been out of balance for many years. He himself put down the start of his anxiety attacks to an incident as a child when he nearly died. A deep-seated fear of impending disaster had hung over him since then, and yet he was himself surprised to note how often he had made his way towards situations which actively courted risk, enjoying only those sports which involved an element of danger. In his career and personal life, however, he was as though paralyzed, frightened to embark on any long-term relationship and unable to develop his obvious talents in any particular direction. He felt, as he put it, 'as though I am stagnating', a condition Water most fears. His Water energy, far from helping his life to flow freely, had become frozen, immobilizing him behind a screen of anxieties.

Treatment helped restore the flow of energy to this element. It was now able to give his spine the support it needed, returning flexibility to his rigid back, and releasing it from pain. His increased sense of balance helped reduce his underlying anxiety, giving him the reassuring feeling that life could not now overwhelm him. Secure in this knowledge, he felt free to venture forward again, and started to make the necessary changes to his work and private life which were eventually to lead him to a good relationship and more fulfilling work.

Water's deeply felt need in some way to challenge itself almost to the point of disaster does not have to play itself out in terms of physical risk alone, as in the case of this patient. Water people may also find themselves in situations which provide a sense of emotional danger, perhaps by choosing a partner of whom they are never quite sure, for such a relationship will bring with it that element of uncertainty with which Water is at heart truly at home.

THE QUALITIES OF THE ELEMENTS
The particular gifts of the elements
Each element holds within itself the knowledge of those particular gifts of which it is the unique trustee, and to which no other element has the key. The following are some of them:

- For Wood, it is the ability to start, for Fire the ability to relate, for Earth the ability to sustain, for Metal the ability to extract and for Water the ability to rejoin.

- Wood looks to others for structure, Fire for love, Earth for comfort, Metal for respect and Water for reassurance.

- Wood acts and gives us hope, Fire relates and gives us joy, Earth supports and gives us understanding, Metal judges and gives us significance and Water survives and unifies.

- Anger strengthens Wood, joy lights Fire's way, sympathy supports Earth, grief purifies Metal and fear helps Water evade danger.

- Water and Earth are the two elements apparently most susceptible to being overwhelmed by life, for, in their differing ways, both have a sense of deep insecurity when their energy is out of balance. And yet in reality these are the two elements least likely to go under. Wood can wither at its roots, Fire can burn itself out and Metal stifle itself. No similar force can destroy Earth or Water. Earthquakes and tempests can buffet the surfaces of land and sea, yet leave undisturbed the depths beneath.

The fears of each element

- Wood's terror is that it will be denied growth, a bud forever closed.
- Fire's terror is that it might never know what love is, its heart eternally cold.
- Earth's terror is that it will be left unquickened, unable to bear fruit.
- Metal's terror is that it is only ever a breath's-breadth away from death.
- Water's terror is that it will be hemmed in, unable to flow and drown in itself.

The challenges for each element

At the moment of death:

- Wood would like to say, 'I gave the world more shape'
- Fire would like to say, 'I made the world a happier place'
- Earth would like to say, 'I gave the world greater understanding'
- Metal would like to say, 'I gave the world more meaning'
- Water would like to say, 'I survived'

CHAPTER 3

COMPONENTS OF FIVE ELEMENT DIAGNOSIS

The patient-practitioner relationship
The Traditional Diagnosis (TD)
TD checklist of questions
Note-taking
Sensory and emotional signatures
Training our senses
The level of imbalance
The causes of disease

THE PATIENT-PRACTITIONER RELATIONSHIP

Now we must carry the understanding we have gained from this brief journey around the elements forward into the practice room, treating these five elemental forces with the awe we reserve for the deepest expressions of life and allowing some of this awe to guide our hand each time we lift the needle. Deep at the heart of that elusive quality which we all look for in those to whom we turn for help is the rare quality of compassion. Both the Latin origin of the word ('feeling with'), and its sister Greek word, sympathy, express that precious ability which is one person's capacity to make another's experiences their own. It demands much of the listener or confidant, for it asks that, for the time of the encounter, he or she steps outside the narrow range of his own needs and experiences, and makes himself for a time a receptacle for those of another. For each patient, the practitioner must endeavour to open up a channel of communication enabling that patient to express his being openly and without fear of judgement or incomprehension.

If we were able to find that help from within our own resources or our own network of support we would not be looking outwards to an acupuncturist. To have taken that difficult first step of making an appointment with an unknown person is an act of faith, requiring courage, and for some people very great courage. Then to find that act of faith rewarded only by an inappropriate or inadequate response is a bitter disappointment. Not to be understood when one is crying out for understanding is a terrible blow, for it makes us feel all the more isolated.

One image may help to illustrate the nature of the patient/practitioner relationship and the step-by-step progress of treatment, and that is one I take from nature. I see successful treatment much like the slow unfolding of a flower, petal by petal. At the heart of the five element practice lies the all-important contact between patient and practitioner. The moment of first contact, when the practitioner meets the patient for the first time and starts to get to know him/her, creates the bud out of which grows all that follows.

This first meeting yields information which will form the basis of a tentative diagnosis and will in turn lead us to select our patient's first treatment based on this diagnosis. The petals of our flower unfold a little more at each encounter. We will assess how this treatment has affected our patients when they return for their second treatment, and we will add this information to our preliminary diagnosis, seeing it either as further confirmation of our initial diagnosis or as modifying it in one way or another. And so the flower grows from petal to petal.

It is important to view treatment in this organic way, seeing it as something which grows only if nurtured by the warmth of the interaction between patient and practitioner. The diagnosis made and the treatment selected fall on fallow ground if not fertilized in this way. The secret to successful five element practice lies in that delicate point of contact between these two people, the one seeking help, the other seeking to help.

Each encounter offers a unique challenge, demanding of us that we approach this person with fresh eyes and leave behind as we enter the practice room all that may detract from the focused spotlight we play upon our patients.

THE TRADITIONAL DIAGNOSIS (TD)

An example of the list of questions to which we need answers from our patient is given below. You should not go through these questions as if you are asking the patient to fill in a questionnaire, but choose an order which feels natural. Ideally, the TD should last 1½–2 hours, and will include the Physical Diagnosis (see Chapter 4). If it is not possible to give a patient this amount of time, the TD should be continued the next time you see the patient until you gradually collect together the answers you need to get a good idea of your patient's life, his/her problems and what his/her needs are.

The important thing about a TD is not to spend too much time on concentrating on the physical problems the patient tells you about. Since most patients initially tend to think acupuncture is only there to treat physical issues, we need to move them gently on to talk about their emotional problems, since we know that these are often the cause of their physical problems. You are not doing a good TD if you find that you have spent most of the time concentrating on physical problems, but have really not got a good understanding of your patient's emotional needs.

We need to gather as much information about our patient as we can as quickly as we can so that we start to build up a picture of their life that puts the problems with which they are coming to us for help into as wide a context as possible. But we must do this sensitively. There is a great skill in guiding the TD along lines which help fill in this context. It should not be a bald list of questions and answers, but should provide us with enough detailed information to pinpoint the areas of a patient's life which may be where the real problems lie.

The crucial factor in guiding a good TD in the right direction is not to use this list as a checklist we tick off, item by item in the order given, but to remember that we need to be alert to any sign that our questioning has touched upon a sensitive area, indicating that there is something significant to be explored here which points us in another direction. The important thing is to note that here is something we need to look at in greater detail, and to make a quick decision as to whether to probe more deeply here or to return to this later on.

It is the patient's answers which reveal some hesitation or disturbance which should be interpreted as hidden cries for help, and we must always show that we have heard these cries. Patients base the trust they feel in their practitioner on their ability to interpret such signs accurately, or, like snails withdrawing their antennae, withdraw into their own emotional shells as soon as they sense that something they are hinting at as being important to them has not been heard or has been ignored.

TD CHECKLIST OF QUESTIONS

- Name/age/date of birth/address/contact details
- Why is the patient coming for treatment?
    - Physical problems?
    - Emotional stresses?

- Relationships
  - Living situation: Living with parent(s), partner, alone?
  - Are they happy with their living situation?
  - How is their relationship with partner/husband/wife?
  - How is their relationship with their parent(s)?
- Any children?
  - If yes, does the patient find it easy being a parent?
  - If no children, did the patient want children, want them in the future?
  - (For women: Any miscarriages/terminations? If so, how has this affected them?)
- Occupation
  - What does the patient do?
  - Does the patient enjoy his/her work?
  - Why did the patient choose this kind of work?
- Plans for the future
  - What would the patient like to change in his/her life? Have they any plans to do this?
- Physical problems
  - Full medical history
  - Any major illnesses?
  - Any surgery?
  - Any chronic complaints?
  - On medication? If so, what medication and for what?
- Sleep
  - What is their sleep like?
  - When do they fall asleep/wake up?
- Bowels
  - Diarrhoea/constipation?

- Bladder
  - Frequency/any pain?
- Perspiration
  - Excessive?
  - Which part of the body?
- For women: periods
  - Regular/painful?
  - In menopause?
- Smoking
  - Do they smoke?
  - For how many years?
  - How many cigarettes a day?
- Recreational drugs
  - Now?
  - In the past?
- Time of day (favourite and least favourite)
- Season (favourite and least favourite)
- Climate (favourite and least favourite)
- Physical Diagnosis
  - Pulse-taking
  - Blood pressure
  - Three jiao
  - Alarm points
  - Centre pulse
  - Akabane test
  - Look in patient's eye for possession (see Chapter 7)

NOTE-TAKING

Ideally everything the patient says is important, and some people therefore like to use a tape recorder to record every word. I dislike this habit, because nobody likes to think that there is a permanent record of what they have said stored somewhere. The presence of a tape recorder is therefore likely to place an obstacle between patient and practitioner, much as though the patient could be talking to a journalist, and will show all the caution any of us would have about revealing details of our personal life in such a situation. In any case, the practicality of listening to up to two hours of tape for every new patient makes it unlikely that the practitioner will ever have the time to play back the tape in any useful way.

We obviously have to take some notes, and we get better at noting down what is important information (the date of major surgery, the medication the patient is on, for example), as well as any key emotional landmarks we have detected as areas of concern. You need never worry if you have forgotten to write down something you later consider is important. Just ask the patient the next time to fill you in a little more about this. They will be only too delighted that you are showing sufficient interest in them to have remembered such details. Often the second time of asking reveals different aspects because by now we hope your patient trusts you enough to open up a little more. The fact that you are interested enough to ask for more information gives the patient proof that you are hearing what they are telling you, and deepens the relationship between you. How much you write down will, with experience, gradually be honed down to only the most significant details, and each practitioner will learn to develop their own particular form of shorthand as they listen to their patients.

We should never sit there with an i-Pad or other electronic device on our lap or desk, tapping away whilst the patient talks. It is essential that we always maintain as much eye contact with our patient as we can, whilst managing to jot down the odd note at the same time. This is something I have got better at doing over the years. But be warned, you should always read back your notes immediately after the patient has left, otherwise you may not be able to decipher your handwriting. Your writing may become more and more undecipherable because of the speed at which you need to write, and you need to use your memory to fill in the blanks quickly afterwards.

This is yet another skill of the many skills a five element acupuncturist needs to develop.

SENSORY AND EMOTIONAL SIGNATURES

It is only once we have laid the groundwork for our diagnosis by taking the first steps in establishing a good relationship with our patient that our diagnosis can move on to the next stage, in which we look for the manifestations of the different elements in our patient and chart their relative balance or imbalance. The elements, and our guardian element in particular, will reflect any stress they are suffering by disturbances in the energies flowing through us. Signals of distress will be sent from the organs deep within us through their meridian pathways to emerge on the surface of the skin as information our senses of sight, hearing and smell and our emotional antennae can pick up. Information revealing what are the four 'diagnostic legs of the stool', those of colour, sound, smell and emotion, is supplemented by a specific form of pulse diagnosis and by other more peripheral information, which together form the basis of the first diagnosis. This initial diagnosis is corroborated or amended as we assess the effects of each treatment, and add to this the deepening layers of understanding which each encounter with a patient brings.

The characteristic signatures of the different elements have been charted since the earliest times. Thus the colour red is seen as an imprint of the Heart and Small Intestine upon us, the sound shouting that of the Gall Bladder and Liver. The particular shadings of this red or of this shouting voice provide very precise diagnostic information about the organs' state of balance. A little less or more of red, or a little less or more of a shouting tone, will indicate either deficiency or excess energy flowing through the meridians. The ability to translate accurately the sensory information we receive into the language of the elements and then transform this into appropriate treatment for our patients forms the very heart of five element diagnosis.

The signals the organs send to the surface of the skin evoke an immediacy of sensory response in us, and because of this immediacy become powerful diagnostic tools when our skills are honed appropriately. One of their advantages is that they can bypass some of the complications our minds can strew in our way. They reflect accurately the level of balance of the organs, and the information they provide will be checked and re-checked before, during and after treatment, as the changes which treatment brings about are assessed.

A five element diagnosis involves filtering sensory impressions over an extended period of time. It requires skill and patience to distinguish the dominant diagnostic indicators from amongst all the signals the other elements within us are sending out. This always takes time, but we get somewhat quicker at it as we build up our repertoire of pointers to the elements. The sensory information we receive, and which we learn to interpret with increasing accuracy, is very sensitive, revealing the slightest deviation from a state of balance.

The emotional signals we all send out can be suppressed, and require interpreting at a deeper level than the other sensory signals. Life may teach us from our earliest days that it is safer to hide some of our vulnerabilities, and to do so we have learnt to a lesser or greater extent to don masks to survive. We smile when we want to cry or shout to hide our fear. To unearth the true emotion behind a patient's mask demands a further focus to the diagnosis, the development of a caring and trusting relationship between patient and practitioner in which the patient feels confident enough to reveal themselves as they are, without fear of judgement or misunderstanding. The practice room has to become a safe place where patients can be encouraged to allow the smile to fade as the fear or anger can at last allow itself true expression, the voice to deepen as grief is permitted to appear.

TRAINING OUR SENSES

'Lose your minds and come to your senses', we were always being told by my teacher, J.R. Worsley. The social veneer we all place around us has to some extent to be stripped away to allow us to develop our senses and be in direct contact with our own and others' emotions. This is by no means an easy task for any of us. It requires a form of reconnection with the purest, most profound parts of ourselves, a truly wondrous experience for those brave enough to pass through what can be seen as a rite of initiation into our deepest selves.

When we first embark on our studies, the elements as they express themselves in each one of us are unknown quantities to us. As their characteristics become more familiar to us, we grow to perceive them more clearly and develop ways of storing all the parcels of information we have gleaned, ready to be retrieved as we make our next diagnosis. We learn to detect the presence of the elements more and more quickly in ourselves and in those we encounter, as we build up our repertoire of all these elemental signposts.

What, then, are we looking for once we have started to train our senses and look within ourselves in this way? First, we must start to build up a catalogue of references accumulated patient by patient which will act as templates against which to compare the sensory information we receive from each new patient who comes to us. Once we have gained a clear view of the colour white on a patient's face, for example, we will store this memory away under the category Metal in our reference catalogue, and take it out to help us with the next patient whose skin has the same pointers to a similar colour on her.

Similarly, a voice once heard and attributed to one or other element will find its echo in that of another patient, and, by a series of comparisons between the different timbres of voices we have heard at different times, will gradually filter itself down to a particular element. Even if we are initially unsure how to categorize that patient in sensory terms, changes resulting from treatment will gradually emphasize one or other colour or emotion, and this will help our diagnosis.

The four diagnostic indicators, if assessed appropriately, will offer us accurate information about the state of balance of a patient's energy. In the case of Wood, for example, we will assess whether the green colour is a balanced expression of the Liver and Gall Bladder's activity, or whether the tone of voice contains excess anger, or, just as unbalanced an expression, an inability to express anger, which we call a lack of anger. Excess or deficiency of any element's energies are both as detrimental to our balance as each other. If excess anger is displayed, there may be unbridled expression of that element's needs. If appropriate expression of anger is suppressed, there will be denial of the existence of anger. It is our ability to maintain our balance within the range of what is appropriate in any one situation which constitutes balance in acupuncture terms.

Acupuncturists have to learn these diagnostic skills, exercising them much as a tennis player exercises on the tennis court. We are initially not skilled in observing the changing colours on people's faces or detecting the changing smells on the body, or the changing sounds of the voices as one or other official shows its unease. Nor may we be sensitive enough to detect emotional changes, or even to be sufficiently aware of the emotions that are flying around us, so immersed are we often in our own problems. We therefore have to spend time re-learning a baby's instinctive assessment of emotional mood and instinctive response to that mood, learning, too, to discount any shadows of our own which we throw over our patients.

There are other indicators to an element in addition to the information which our senses yield, for everything we do, being a product of the elements' work, reveals their complex interrelationships within each one of us to a sensitive observer. But none of these will offer the reliability of information which our senses can provide once they have been properly trained and exercised. These other sources of information will be of use in helping support our diagnosis in cases where the sensory information has given us an insufficiently firm foundation. For example, people of different elements have a tendency to approach things in different ways, to act in different ways, to make decisions in different ways, even to dress in different ways. The information we glean from such observations is initially less reliable than those provided by our senses, but becomes increasingly significant with experience. We will also learn gradually to become aware of the responses within us to a particular element, one perhaps making us slightly tenser, another more relaxed, one drawing us to it, another demanding that we give it space.

Tiny shifts in the balance of energy as a result of treatment also become easier to detect with practice, and may be overlooked to start with. Observing a muddy yellow change take on a more golden glow takes experience to perceive, as our eyes train themselves to see ever finer gradations of colour. The other senses have to be trained, too, and we have to work hard at this, looking carefully at patient after patient in this way. Only when we have seen a greyish-white colour shift to a purer white do we begin to understand what a healthy Metal colour is, or when an exceedingly high-pitched laugh becomes more subdued understand what Fire in balance sounds like. In effect, all practitioners have to train themselves to develop a musician's sharp ears, a painter's sharp eyes and a cook's sharp sense of smell. We also have to develop ever more acute sensitivity to emotional signals.

What the acupuncturist sees is rarely the elements in all their strength and vigour, as they express themselves in a healthy person – and this begs the question of whether any of us can indeed ever be truly balanced – but some distortion, an emotion hidden, a colour exaggerated. In our diagnosis we are looking for what jars, since the inappropriate stands out strongly, beckoning us to take note. If I am unhappy but smile, or talk of my loved ones with sadness in my voice, or describe unemotionally events of great trauma, my listener, if he is acute enough, will be aware of something amiss. Event and emotion do not appear to match. Some slippage has occurred, some shift, so that what is below the surface no longer matches what is above. A distortion of some kind has detached the emotion from what it should be an expression of. The greater the detachment, the more this is evidence of some fundamental state of imbalance.

It is in detecting such inconsistencies, and then charting their progress as treatment attempts to correct them, that the skills of five element practice lie.

THE LEVEL OF IMBALANCE
The three levels of the human being, our body, our mind and our soul, each have their own needs and express their imbalances in different ways. Those of the soul, emerging from the depths within us, are the most important to address, since our inner being shapes how we cope with whatever physical distresses we have to contend with.

All treatment, being addressed at the patient as a whole, touches all levels and no one level can be treated without the others being affected. In the Western world we have made more discrete entities of ourselves, sending our souls, as it were, to church, our minds to our psychiatrists and our bodies to hospital. In acupuncture, on the other hand, we do not view one organ or one part of our body or soul as something which can or should be treated on its own. Thus each treatment, affecting as it does the person as a whole, will have some resonance for each of the three levels. Some treatments, though, may have a more specific focus to address specific needs, such as those where we have diagnosed that the patient's spirit is very low, for example. But even the apparently humblest point provides a connection to the deepest level of our being, and this deepest level spreads its influence upon the surface of our body.

By diagnosing the depth of our patient's imbalance and endeavouring to assess whether we feel a patient needs their inner spirit warming or strengthening, we are making an assessment of the level of this patient's imbalance. Those who are dealing robustly with even the most traumatic onslaughts of life can be said to have a strong spirit, and we can diagnose these patients as being out of balance at a more superficial level, that of the mind. The most superficial of all imbalances is that of the mere body, the physical level, but here, too, the severity of a physical imbalance will impact immediately upon the deeper levels so that by the time the patient reaches us the imbalance, if severe, will have spread to these levels, too. If, for example, a person has been in a car crash and suffers whiplash injury, the worry about how long she will take to recover will affect her mental processes and eventually also her spirit if the injury persists and she feels unable to carry on her normal work. And, too, the trauma of the crash itself, even if no injury is sustained, will have affected her emotionally, so that she may have trouble afterwards in driving a car.

Each time we select a point we do so not merely for its energetic function, which is to stabilize the energies flowing between the officials, but also for what we call its spirit, and we are doing this on the basis of an assessment of the level of the patient's imbalance on that day.

THE CAUSES OF DISEASE

Traditionally acupuncturists have drawn upon a list of what are called internal and external causes of disease, and I give below the one I inherited. I have seen different variants, but all are approximately the same. The list is considered to cover the total range of all those causes which can eventually lead to imbalance in a human being.

External causative factors
- Humidity
- Dampness
- Dryness
- Fire
- Heat
- Cold
- Wind

Internal causative factors
- Anger
- Joy
- Worry
- Grief
- Fear
- Anxiety
- Constitutional and inherited factors

Miscellaneous
- Toxicity
- Pollution
- Radiation
- Diet/lifestyle

The two main groups are those for internal and external causes. The small third list, which is tagged on rather unhappily, covers anything not already included under the main groups. There is, however, a good case for incorporating the items listed as miscellaneous within these two main groupings. Toxicity, pollution and radiation could then be regarded as external causes, with diet/lifestyle straddling both groups.

It is interesting to note the emphasis which different branches of acupuncture place on one or other category. It will be obvious that five element acupuncture predominantly emphasizes the internal aspects, which include within them, though in a slightly wider arc, the five great emotional signatures of the elements. Although they are here listed as seven, it is easy to see how fear and anxiety can be brought together under the umbrella of Water, with constitutional and inherited factors being a factor of all the elements. The external aspects, too, have each their clear association with an element, with the Fire element covering both fire and heat, and Earth both humidity and dampness.

External causes will also impact upon our inner life, for example if we are mugged and are frightened of going out alone, just as internal causes will affect the outside, for example if our anger makes us unable to function at work. Although other branches of acupuncture place much greater emphasis upon the external causes, these can also provide additional diagnostic information in five element acupuncture. For example, we need to know the climate, season and time of day a patient feels in or out of balance in, since this will point to an external cause of imbalance.

It can be seen that five element acupuncture tends to work from inside outwards whilst other branches of acupuncture tend to work from outside inwards. All, if based upon valid principles which chime with what we know of the human being, will be equally effective, meeting as it were in the middle, since both inside and outside have to be in harmony. The distinctions between all these categories must therefore always be blurred, but as broad categories they describe useful differences of emphasis.

CHAPTER 4

Secondary Diagnostic Information

Pulse-taking
Blood pressure
Three jiao
Alarm points
Centre pulse
Akabane test

PULSE-TAKING

Apart from the information we gain from observing colour, sound, smell and emotion, we can obtain additional information which can help us make a more accurate diagnosis. From Western medicine we know that the pulse at the wrist, and elsewhere on the body where it is palpable, conveys information about the functioning of the heart. In acupuncture terms it also tells us much about the other officials as well as the heart. Different methods of pulse-taking and pulse interpretation have been developed by different acupuncture traditions over the years.

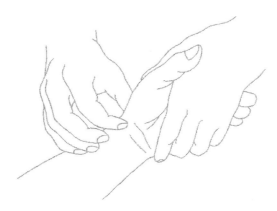

J.R. Worsley taught us that as we palpate each pulse we should ask each official, 'Small Intestine, what do you want today?', 'Heart, what do you want today?' These questions remove pulse-taking from the mere physical recording of a pulse beat, and place it firmly at the deeper level of the spirit. Here the instrument of nature we must become opens up a channel of communication through which the patient's officials speak their needs. We are feeling for the quality of the pulses, and the contact established bypasses the mind's attempts to think its way to an interpretation of the pulse, allowing the pulse to speak directly to the practitioner's spirit. Feeling a thing is so, with our spirit, is very different from thinking a thing is so, with our mind. This is why it is so important not to dwell too long on a pulse reading, for the spirit's perceptions are very immediate (we see anger or joy in a flash), whereas the mind may need to ponder over what it sees.

Such is the power of the mind, too, that it is also possible to think your way to changing a pulse reading merely by allowing your mind to entertain another thought. You can take two very different pulse readings if your state of mind changes. Doubt can alter a pulse reading, as can somebody else's suggestion. Calming the mind and spirit before taking a pulse reading can therefore form an essential part of our practice, enabling us to clear away some of the thoughts which cloud us. Shutting the eyes is a useful way of helping a student develop that inner concentration and stillness which allows the pulses to talk deeply to us. Later on, this becomes less necessary, because, as all those who meditate know, keeping contact with the outside world whilst in contact with our inner world is one of the deepest forms of meditation.

How to take pulses

The practitioner holds the patient's hand with both hands so that the hand is held securely. This close contact also forms part of the five element practitioner's emphasis upon the importance of touch as a diagnostic tool and as a way of transmitting comfort and support to the patient. The fingers are placed over the radial artery as shown in the diagram. Whilst taking the pulses, the practitioner also notes the patient's response to touch, as well as the texture and temperature of the patient's skin. As treatment progresses, any changes in these diagnostic indicators will also be added to information gained from changes in pulse picture.

The pulse positions used in five element acupuncture are based on those listed in the Nan Jing, and reached this country by way of Japanese schools of acupuncture. The method of palpation used is to palpate with the tips of the fingers rather than with the pads, as in some other branches of acupuncture.

The pulse positions are as follows:

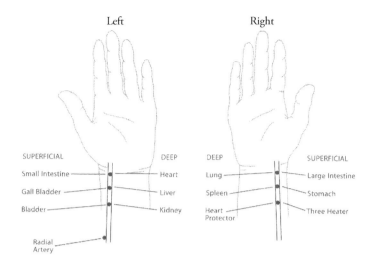

The pulse reading is based on a differentiation between the relative qualities of the pulses, designated as plus, check or minus, and can in principle range from -3 to +3. In practice, however, since nobody is in perfect health, pulse readings are rarely, if ever, check, that is, in balance, nor can one pulse be in balance if the others are not, since all the officials will show stress if one is stressed. A pulse which is read as -1 is more deficient than one of +1, and one of +1 is more in excess than one of -1. Neither + nor - is better than the other, since both represent a deviation from balance, the check pulse. The relative balance of pulses one to another will represent the state of harmony or disharmony within the elements and between the officials.

Example of a pulse notation

Left		Right	
Superficial	*Deep*	*Deep*	*Superficial*
-1	-1	-¾	-¾
-1½	-1½	-1	-1
-2	-2	-2	-2

Using this method of pulse-taking, deficiency in energy is much more frequent than excess energy. The officials predominantly need to be given more energy (tonification method of needling) rather than have energy drained from them (sedation method).

What pulses can tell us

Before treatment starts:

- The presence of the following blocks to treatment:
  - Husband-Wife imbalance
  - Entry-Exit block
- The relative strengths and weaknesses of the officials
- The overall strength and weakness, and therefore the level of imbalance

At the end of treatment:

- Whether the officials' state of balance has improved or not
- Whether there have been changes in the relative strengths and weaknesses of the officials
- Whether any fresh Entry-Exit blocks have occurred

It is important to remember that it can take some time for energy to shift after treatment. Pulses are likely to change significantly as energy slowly moves towards greater balance. A pulse reading at the end of treatment will always therefore be only a temporary reading, and should not be used as a clear indicator of the effectiveness of a particular treatment.

What pulses cannot tell us

- Which element is the guardian element

Overview of the essential requirements for pulse-taking

- Remaining as calm as possible
- Having as uncluttered a mind as possible
- Allowing the fingers to feel and the officials to talk
- Understanding what information pulses can or cannot give us
- Developing the ability to cope with the subjective nature of pulse-taking
- Learning to evaluate appropriately the level of our pulse-taking skills so that we do not develop over-reliance on our pulse readings

BLOOD PRESSURE

The level of a patient's blood pressure is always significant as a general gauge of health, and is the main factor in deciding whether or not to add moxibustion, an essential component of five element practice.

Moxibustion is contraindicated in the following cases:

- If a patient has a high BP, or has a differential of more than 40 between diastolic and systolic pressures. In this case the BP should be taken regularly as treatment progresses to see whether it reverts to within the normal range. Moxibustion can be added if it does so. If a patient is on BP medication, and the BP readings are normal, moxibustion can be introduced very slowly to see whether it affects the BP. If it appears to cause the BP to rise, it should be discontinued. In some cases, moxibustion may help the BP fall as the warming it brings to treatment relaxes stress upon the heart.

- If moxibustion on a specific point is forbidden. For a list of points which are forbidden to moxa, see J.R. Worsley's *The Meridians of Ch'i Energy: Point Reference Guide*.[*]

THREE JIAO

Five element acupuncture uses two main forms of palpation to provide secondary diagnostic information, each of which gives us information about areas of sensitivity on the body. Each also provides information about the state of balance of the different officials, and is a gauge of the progress of treatment. They may sometimes, but more rarely, determine treatment selection. It is expected that imbalances revealing themselves as fluctuations in temperature in the case of the three jiao or tenderness in the case of alarm points will gradually disappear as the officials come into balance with one another.

Palpation of the three jiao helps us assess the balance of the Three Heater as registering in the three areas of the abdomen over which it has control.

---

[*] Worsley, J.R. (1979) *The Meridians of Ch'i Energy: Point Reference Guide*. Maryland: The Traditional Acupuncture Institute, Inc.

Upper jiao	**Above the diaphragm**
Organs of intake	Heart
	Heart Protector
	Lung
Middle jiao	**Above the umbilicus**
Organs of processing	Gall Bladder
	Liver
	Stomach
	Spleen
Lower jiao	**Below the umbilicus**
Organs of elimination	Small Intestine
	Bladder
	Kidney
	Large Intestine

The hand is placed in contact with the skin over the upper, middle and lower jiao in turn, and a reading taken of their relative degree of warmth. The blanket covering the patient should be pulled back a few minutes before taking the reading to ensure that the overall temperature of the body is the same before palpation.

The balance of the three jiao is recorded on a scale of -, ✓ and + as shown in the following example:

    Upper jiao   ✓
    Middle jiao   -
    Lower jiao   ✓

In this example, the middle jiao is cooler to the touch than the upper or lower jiao. This information tells us about the relative balance of the three groups of officials one to another, and helps us assess whether there have been changes as a result of treatment.

We use this diagnostic information to select treatment only if a clear imbalance in one or other of the jiao persists after some period of treatment. For example, if the lower jiao is persistently cooler than the others and we wish to select a CV point for treatment, we may consider using a lower CV point, for example CV 5 or CV 7, to help restore balance to the area in which the Three Heater is showing distress.

ALARM POINTS

A further form of palpation is that relating to what are called alarm points. Each official is seen has having a relationship to a particular acupuncture point which will show that official's state of balance by its sensitivity to pressure. The alarm point may become tender if the official to which it relates is under stress. It is not uncommon for patients to report pain or tenderness and locate it precisely on an alarm point.

To assess this, each alarm point is palpated in turn by finger pressure and the patient's reactions recorded. As treatment progresses, a change in sensitivity at one or other point will indicate a greater state of balance.

Use in treatment

Sometimes it may be appropriate to use an alarm point in treatment. For example, it might be appropriate to use the alarm point of the Large Intestine, XI 25 (St 25), to treat an Earth patient who is constipated and on whom this point is tender. In certain cases, this would also be a suitable point to do on a patient of another element, but only after extensive treatment on his/her own guardian element has not helped the patient. In the same way, we might consider using CV 12 if we have a patient with a persistently cold middle jiao.

List of alarm points

Organ	Point	
Heart	CV 14	
Small Intestine	CV 4	
Bladder	CV 3	
Kidney	VII 25 (GB 25)	
Heart Protector	CV 15	
Three Heater	CV 17	Upper jiao
	CV 12	Middle jiao
	CV 7	Lower jiao
	CV 5	Main alarm point for whole Three Heater
Gall Bladder	VII 23 (GB 23)	
	VII 24 (GB 24)	
Liver	VIII 14 (Liv 14)	
Lung	IX 1 (Lu 1)	
Large Intestine	XI 25 (St 25)	
Stomach	CV 12	
Spleen	VIII 13 (Liv 13)	

CENTRE PULSE

When palpated, the umbilical (centre) pulse should beat in the centre of the umbilicus. If its beat is off-centre, it will be as though the patient is being thrown constantly to one side or another, much like a top spinning a little out of control.

The position of the centre pulse is recorded as follows. In this example, the pulse is said to be slightly north-east of centre.

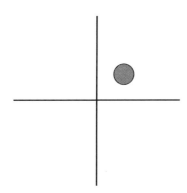

Palpating the centre pulse

The thumb and first two fingers are inserted gently into the umbilicus and pressed down firmly until the pulse is located. It may help to ask the patient to breathe in as you do so as this helps the muscles relax. If the pulse is off-centre, as in the example above, it is palpated into position by placing the palms of the hands on the stomach and pressing both thumbs down behind the pulse, stroking it firmly back towards the centre. The thumbs must press a fold of the skin and not ride over the pulse. This is done by exerting strong, but not uncomfortable pressure, until the pulse beats at the centre of the umbilicus again. It may take a few manipulations to get it centred properly and the patient can also be shown how to correct it. This is an excellent way of involving a patient in his/her treatment.

A centre pulse will usually correct itself with treatment over time, but an initial correction will speed treatment. This correction should be done as part of the Physical Diagnosis during the initial TD (see Chapter 3).

AKABANE TEST

The relative balance of energy passing along the left and right meridians also needs to be checked, and corrected where necessary. This is done by means of what is called an Akabane test. This test is named after a Japanese acupuncturist who discovered the importance of ensuring that the energy flowing along the paired meridians should be relatively in balance. Akabane imbalances can often be the cause of persistent left- or right-sided symptoms. If these occur or recur at any stage during treatment, the Akabanes should be checked again.

The test is carried out, and corrections made, as part of the Physical Diagnosis during the initial TD (see Chapter 3). Any corrections should be done after the centre pulse has been corrected, since an uncentred pulse may affect the Akabane readings.

Procedure

Before the sensitivity of the points is checked, the procedure should be demonstrated to patients to reassure them that the taper will not touch the skin, and that the heat they feel is the point warming up. They should be told to say immediately they feel any warmth, since points once warmed become hot very quickly.

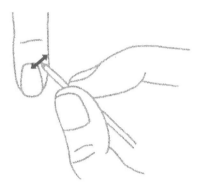

All the nail points on hand and feet are marked, using the medial nail point of the small toe as the Kidney point. A lighted taper is then used to warm the points in turn. The hand holding the taper should be steadied against the couch or the patient's body and the patient's toe or finger should be held firmly. When testing the hands, both of the patient's hands can be placed on the abdomen and the test carried out by moving easily from one to the other, rather than walking round the couch. The sequence followed should always be the same to ensure that the procedure flows smoothly. For example, readings on the hand can be taken from the thumb to the little finger and on the foot from the big to the little toe.

The taper is held just above the point and passed over each pair of nail points in turn, first on the left, then on the right. Each pass over a point is counted. The pass should be at a 45° angle over the corner of the nail, and the taper must pass directly over the point. Care should be taken to ensure that it is held at the same distance from the point and that the angle and length of pass is the same for each pair of points. Once the patient indicates that the point is hot, the taper should be removed immediately and the point pressed firmly to disperse the heat.

If the point warms up after 2 passes on the left and 3 on the right, this is recorded as a reading of ⅔. Each pair of readings should be recorded in turn, and after all are completed the readings should be examined to see whether there is a sufficiently marked difference between one side and the other on any pair to warrant correction. A difference of more than one-third is considered an imbalance. A reading of ⅕ indicates that the meridian on the left has five times more energy passing through it than on the right. The lower the count, the more energy is flowing through the meridian on that side.

Feet are often colder than hands, and it is usual for the count to be higher on the feet. A count of 10–20 passes on the feet and 3–10 on the hands is about average. If counts are consistently much higher than these, there is probably a problem with the technique used. The taper may be too far from the point, or the passes over the point may be too slow or too wide.

Treatment to correct imbalances

For each meridian showing an imbalance, the junction point on the deficient side (the side with the highest count) should be tonified and the reading rechecked. If an imbalance remains, the source point on the deficient side is then tonified. If this still fails to correct the imbalance, the paired points should be rechecked again after about 5–6 treatments to see whether the imbalance has corrected itself. If not, it can be corrected again using the same procedure.

Sometimes the correction treatment can lead to an imbalance the other way. This can be ignored, as it is only temporary.

It is likely that most imbalances between paired meridians will in any case correct themselves spontaneously as treatment progresses and a healthy balance to the flow of energy is restored. Akabane corrections are a way of speeding up this process, and help to reduce the stress caused by tension between the two sides of a meridian. There are, however, cases where such spontaneous correction is unlikely, for example if someone suffers serious injury to one side of the body, such as a stroke. Here it may be necessary to make repeated corrections to help restore balance.

CHAPTER 5

Treatment

The different stages of treatment
The spacing of treatments
Assessing the effects of treatment
The Law of Cure
The patient's role in treatment

THE DIFFERENT STAGES OF TREATMENT

Treatment is carried out by needling and applying moxibustion to acupuncture points which lie at intervals along the meridians associated with the two officials of each element. A treatment will pass through several stages, each fulfilling a particular aim. The first stage covers the first few treatments, and consists in selecting points which help us assess the state of our patient's energy and then start building it up slowly. In this stage of treatment, we select points which address the patient's element directly, but as gently as possible, since a patient's energy is quite volatile and sensitive at the start of treatment and will only accept the gentlest nudge to start with. We are also using these initial treatments to find out whether we are focusing our treatment on the right segment of the five element cycle.

Each treatment asks questions of the element we have chosen by offering it help and then leaving us to assess whether it wants this help, and, if so, whether it is the right help we are offering. If we are not addressing the element in need, there will be no response at all or a less emphatic response than if we focus the treatment exactly where it is needed. It is in deciphering correctly the nature of such responses that much of the diagnostic skill of five element acupuncture lies. It is therefore important to ask questions of the treatment appropriate for its different stages.

We have many different groupings of acupuncture points available to us to help us move on from stage to stage in this way. These provide us with a solid repertoire of points from which to select our initial treatments. All contribute to determining the state of balance of the officials in question and then strengthening them where we find weaknesses. Once the initial foundations have been secured, treatment moves to the next stage in which we address the officials more directly and forcefully now that we feel confident that we are focusing on the right element.

Once on firmer ground in this way, we move on to using points for what we call their spirit. Here we draw on the differing qualities residing in each point. And this is when a practitioner's more individual approach to treatment selection starts to come into play. Here individual points are selected with actions about which there is much discussion. The points we select will be determined largely by the tradition each of us inherits and by our individual interpretation of the significance of the points in relation to our understanding of their location or name, and of the elements to which they belong. Knowledge of the Chinese etymology forming the characters of point names undoubtedly adds to this understanding. But since much debate centres around the translation of the characters, (and we need only compare different point translations to see this), I believe we do ourselves a disservice if we deny ourselves the right to our own interpretation of point meanings within the context of our personal view of the officials. To some extent, then, each of us will nurture our own family of points with which we feel comfortable. We will continue to add new points as we extend our understanding and gain more courage to explore a little further into the unknown territory each new point represents.

When I qualified, I was taught, I think quite brilliantly, to start with the simple, and stay within the small circumference of familiar points, only venturing into the wider world of point selection as my confidence grew, and more importantly my understanding of the profound depths contained within each point deepened. I learnt to approach new points with the caution they deserved, and where I was in doubt or unsure I retreated back to more familiar terrain. We were given clear ground rules with which even a newly qualified acupuncturist could feel safe. Such teaching helped demystify the whole area of point selection, removing much of the uncertainties I see some practitioners now experiencing.

I have concluded that, beyond the first treatments, the order in which we select individual points which are on the element we are treating and the nature of the points we select does not appear to be as important as the effect created by the constant strengthening and balancing of the officials by selecting point after point on these officials. It is as though each time we address an element through one of its points a further brick is added to reinforce the foundation of that element. Provided we build up a solid foundation in this way, and do this appropriately floor by floor, it may well not matter whether we start with the kitchen or the hallway, as it were.

It is important, therefore, to encourage ourselves not to see the success of treatment as residing in points in themselves, but in the strengthening of the elemental structure as a whole which we are helping put together. Treatment is a cumulative process. If we see a point as each time offering the officials something slightly different, each being a little instruction to them to adjust their energy in some way, then what we must beware of is not confusing our patients' energy with too many of these instructions. Better by far to return regularly to the security of simple treatments to allow the officials a breathing space in which to strengthen themselves quietly. If not, we may hammer them too hard, and they will grow tired. We know that they will sometimes need powerful treatments which force them to change direction, but after these they always need time to readjust and recoup.

We should always remind ourselves that the effects of treatment are long term and that it usually takes time for improvements to make themselves felt. Each treatment shifts a patient's energy slightly, but not so drastically as to unbalance them. We must therefore not be impatient on our patients' behalf, but give treatment time to take effect. We should always use the least possible number of points so that the interference in our patient's energy which each treatment signifies is as brief and as effective as possible. This will help to reinforce our understanding of the power of simple treatment, and will help deter us from offering unnecessarily complex combinations of points whose purpose we are unclear about. Simplicity and purity of intent are all.

THE SPACING OF TREATMENTS

The aim of treatment is to return a patient's energy to a state of sufficient balance to remove the need for treatment except as a form of preventive medicine or as a continuing support. Since every intervention with the needle interferes in however slight a way with a patient's control of their own energy, we want them to be in a position to reassert this control. Control has to be handed back to our patient gradually, but as quickly as possible. If not, there is a danger that a patient may become dependent on both treatment and practitioner. This can happen with any replacement therapy, a description which can also be applied to acupuncture. It is therefore our responsibility to ensure that we only usurp the patient's own role of being master of his/her energies for as brief a time as possible to allow for changes to take place and then be maintained.

How frequent treatment should be is a matter of professional judgement, and regulating its frequency appropriately is an art in itself. Learning to gauge how often a particular patient should come is a skill we gradually acquire.

Unbalanced energies take time to rebalance themselves. All patients require frequent treatment to start with, from a minimum of once a week for most patients, or even more frequently for those who are very out of balance. How long these weekly or more frequent treatments should continue will depend on improvements in the patient's health. As soon as there have been positive changes which remain constant, probably within 6–8 weeks of the start of treatment, treatment should be extended to once every two weeks, and so on by incremental stages to once every few months and then seasonally, where appropriate.

Patients will themselves contribute to a decision on the spacing of treatment. In the early stages they may not be sufficiently in tune with their own energy to perceive changes. As treatment progresses, however, their self-awareness grows and after a few treatments they will themselves feel when their energy drops or whether treatment can be spaced out further. There will also be times when patients need to come more frequently because of changes they are going through or some crisis in their life. At others, treatment can be spaced more widely.

How much longer patients will choose to continue will depend on how they view their treatment. For those who see treatment as providing a support through a lifetime of changes, it becomes an accompaniment to a patient's journey of self-development. For others, who regard it as helping them to balance or as addressing a particular symptom or issue, it will be a finite process. These patients will stop treatment once this objective is achieved.

Below are some guidelines for helping us judge how to space treatments. Optimum spacing of treatment is based on the following:

- The extent to which treatment is helping restore and maintain balance.

- How seriously ill our patient is: the more seriously ill, the more frequent the need for treatment. No seriously ill patient will get well if given treatment once a month, or even initially only once a week.

- Whether our patient requires constant support through a period of change in their lives, irrespective of whether they are improving or not. Here we have to gauge whether our patient should be encouraged to take responsibility themselves for these changes, or whether the support we can give is essential for them.

ASSESSING THE EFFECTS OF TREATMENT

Patients may come to treatment with many different expectations. For one person, the removal of some physical pain may be all they wish to achieve from their treatment. Another will regard their treatment as supporting major life changes. Some may wish for instantaneous transformation from imbalance to balance, from pain to the absence of pain in one treatment, and have to learn to deal with the inevitable disappointment when unrealistic hopes such as these are dashed. For others, the concern the practitioner shows them is enough in itself to make them feel a little better and return for further treatment with hope in their heart. And this hope alone will help alleviate the weight of their symptoms slightly, which is why patients will often say they feel better just for talking their problems through.

We all have different pain thresholds, too, and different perceptions of what we find unbearable and what we can tolerate. The same headache will not worry us too much on one day, but becomes too intense if we are unhappy at work. Equally, we will each respond to treatment in our differing ways, some impatient for success, others prepared to give their practitioners time. The different expectations with which we come for treatment will make us view any changes that occur from different angles, one person seeing them as amazingly quick, others finding them too slow. The expectations of patient and practitioner may also not match. Practitioners may judge there to have been significant change, in a case where an imbalance has been so entrenched that the slightest shift must be called a triumph of treatment, whereas the patient may be disappointed that so little has changed.

Practitioners, too, will have their own differing expectations of what the treatment they offer can achieve. Here, too, these may range from the unrealistic to the unnecessarily pessimistic. We may ask ourselves whether we are capable of meeting our patients' expectations. What if we fall short, prove unequal to the task we set ourselves, at its highest level that of helping to transform another's life? All these factors have to be taken into account in gauging the success of treatment from the point of view of both patient and practitioner.

What is interesting is that the deeper the practitioner's understanding of the potential power of treatment becomes, the more effectively the fingers that hold the needle guide this accumulated knowledge towards the point. We call this the practitioner's intention. The experienced practitioner has built up a store of acquired knowledge which the inexperienced has yet to gain. This is why the same point can have two different effects if used by two different practitioners, the one creating change and transformation, where the other yields very little.

The part practitioners' intention plays increases with the development of their understanding of the forces with which they are dealing when a needle contacts a point. The deeper this awareness, the greater the likelihood that the practitioner can address these forces, and tap depths through the treatment which a less aware, less skilled practitioner may deny exist or hesitate to address. A practitioner expecting a point to have a resonance only at the physical level will therefore restrict the effectiveness of that point to that level, whereas another practitioner, aware of the deeper currents which this point has the potential to touch upon, will be able to achieve a level of deeper healing unavailable to the first.

We can never predict what will happen, such is the complexity of each patient's unique response, and practitioner and patient await the outcome of each treatment with a similar degree of anticipation. We owe it to our patients to include hope, but not certainty, in what we offer, to keep our own and our patient's expectations to what experience has shown is possible, and then for both of us to be delighted if these expectations are exceeded.

Each patient will have a unique response to treatment, and it is therefore impossible to predict what these responses will be and decide in advance what the next treatment should be. We will write down some proposals for this treatment based upon how we see the patient as they leave, but these will be modified by what we find on the patient's return. As we get to know our patient better, and our reading of the diagnostic signals improves, our diagnosis will move to an ever deeper level. Our treatments have to keep step with this process, and match each level of diagnosis reached. We call this process treatment planning.

The gauge of the success of treatment will come through observing changes in any of the diagnostic information when the patient returns for his/her next treatment. When treatment is effective, some degree of change in one or other of the diagnostic criteria must occur, ranging from a tiny shift to a profound level of transformation. If nothing appears to have changed, this is just as important information, as it tells us that treatment has not yet been focused correctly. If we do not offer the elements what they are calling for, they respond with a deafening silence, and, by their silence, tell us to direct our attention elsewhere.

Some changes may be obvious only to the practitioner. These can vary from very clear changes, such as a marked improvement in pulse picture or an obvious colour change, to more subtle changes, such as a slight reduction in smell, a slight lightening of mood, a slightly lighter step or a slightly brighter eye. We also have to learn to attune ourselves to the subtle variations in a patient's emotional life to assess the extent to which treatment is also leading to changes at the deeper levels. Here we have verbal feedback from our patients to help us, and this will not merely be that of a patient telling us how they feel. We may find patients starting to talk differently about their work or suddenly making plans for a holiday. Somebody who has felt rather isolated now tells us she has got in touch with some old friends again, or we notice that a treatment has gone by without the patient mentioning the frustration with his wife which has preoccupied him for the past few weeks. All these slight changes, often unnoticed by the patients themselves, indicate some shift. And these shifts, if continuous, are a sign that the patient is moving towards greater balance.

We must work on the principle that the less we treat the better, but only if a patient is improving. The less improvement the patient experiences, the more frequently we need to see them so that we can give ourselves enough time to work out what we are not seeing. It is important to be honest and have the courage to ask patients whether they feel there has been any improvement. If they say no, then we must not be afraid to tell them there is something we have not seen, and that we would like them to come more frequently until we get to the bottom of it. If we pretend that things are going better than they are, our patients will see through us. They often come to us because all else has failed, and they are relieved that we are taking them so seriously that we are prepared to give them so much of our time. No patient with whom I have shared my doubts about the progress of treatment in this way has ever been other than pleased at my honesty. Often they are frightened to tell us that things are not improving in case we give up on them, as many others before us have done.

Other questions to ask ourselves if, despite the above, there is no progress in treatment is whether any of the major blocks may have recurred (see Chapter 7), or whether it is possible that we failed to clear them the first time. There may also be something in a patient's life they are not yet prepared to tell us about, such as some emotional trauma, because they do not feel the practice room has become a safe enough place in which to share such confidences. Their lifestyle may also be hindering treatment without our realizing it, and if we suspect this is so we need to look carefully at our patient's history to see whether there are any indications of what this might be. Are they perhaps regularly drinking too much alcohol or have they got hidden eating problems?

Then there is always the possibility that the patient has more to gain by remaining ill than by getting better. We can often check this by giving them some simple tasks to do, such as walking each day for half an hour or drinking more water, and seeing whether they do this. It is surprising how often some patients will make all sorts of excuses not to do what you have told them to, whilst patients who want to get better will make every effort to cooperate. You are in a no-win situation here. The patient wants you to do all the work, without helping himself or herself. You must seriously consider whether it is worth continuing treatment in such cases, for no treatment can succeed without the patient's willingness to contribute towards its success.

It is rare for treatment to make things worse, except temporarily, as a patient moves through a sometimes uncomfortable phase of adjusting to change. We have our own inbuilt safety mechanisms within us which shield our elements' energies from unwelcome interference, and cry out in no uncertain terms if treatment is pushing us against the flow our life should take. One such cry will express itself in a patient's unwillingness to continue treatment. This is in many, but not all, cases a sign that the practitioner is not reading the diagnostic signals accurately enough to translate them into effective treatment, and this includes an inability to establish a supportive patient-practitioner relationship.

If the elements are not receiving the support from treatment which they are calling for, they will remain uneasy and dissatisfied, and the sensory data the practitioner receives will indicate this. Eventually we learn to recognize more clearly the subtle signals each patient sends out as our senses become more finely attuned, and this will help us make increasingly accurate assessments of the state of balance of the elements.

Change can make itself felt in many ways, and a patient's own perception of change also offers crucial information. Here we have to be careful, for patients will react in very differing ways and their reactions will vary at different stages of treatment. In assessing what patients tell us, we must remember that change can be uncomfortable and may therefore be unwelcome to the patient, so that what may be a necessary jolt turning them in the direction of health may be perceived by them as unpleasant. They may have to feel worse before they feel better, but may not be happy to acknowledge this. Similarly, some patients will be sufficiently aware to welcome any change as a sign of improvement, and be unworried by the fact that their backache is still there because they feel so much better in themselves. Others may pin their assessment of treatment on the continuing presence of the stomach pains, choosing to ignore the fact that their sleep is so much better.

Finally time is on our side. Patients themselves are usually not in a hurry, provided that we have developed a good relationship with them and are honest with them. A five element diagnosis, like all forms of diagnosis, is extremely complex, and requires us to filter sensory and other input over an extended period of time. This will not concern patients if we do not claim quicker results for treatment than we can achieve and do not allow ourselves to be hurried. If we explain to our patients that we need more time to deepen our diagnosis, they are always willing to give us that time because they are grateful for our care and concern. Patients generally welcome the commitment we are showing by dedicating so much time to each of them.

THE LAW OF CURE

A further gauge of the progress of treatment is known as the Law of Cure, a principle of treatment taken from homeopathy.

Often we deal with pressures upon us, whether physical or emotional, by suppressing our reactions to them. We can do this physically if we take medication to treat a condition, for then the illness has often not been allowed to run its natural course, and may be pushed deeper within the body. We can also do this emotionally by hiding what we feel or denying that we feel it. Everything we experience remains within us, particularly if it is unresolved, when it needs to be dealt with in some way if it is not to fester. We all know what it is like to harbour a grudge when the angry feelings, not allowed any outlet, turn in upon ourselves. We can also harbour physical stresses in the same way. An illness suppressed by medication can hide at a deeper level within us, causing further distress.

As acupuncture treatment starts restoring us to balance, it draws these suppressed imbalances out into the open to be dealt with. This process is known as the Law of Cure. According to this law, all imbalances progress to a natural cure along three possible routes as treatment helps the different layers heal themselves:

- From the top of the body downwards
- From inside the body outwards
- In reverse chronological order to the course of the original imbalances

Imbalances gradually drain away, almost as though through the action of gravity, so that they move from deep inside outwards towards the surface and downwards to be expelled from the body, leaving the person whole. During this process, they may also move chronologically backwards along the course they originally took, retracing their steps and allowing body and soul time to heal themselves at each stage of imbalance in turn. Patients may experience a brief reminder of past imbalances, perhaps a headache for a day when they have suffered migraines in the past, or the appearance of a few spots on the body when they have suffered from acne in the past.

Emotionally too, patients may find themselves dreaming of some traumatic event, or re-experiencing for a period the anger or grief which overwhelmed them years ago. These episodes are always brief, and should pass, leaving the patient calmer and more at peace.

Although we must be careful not to alarm patients, it is important to tell them to let us know if they experience any exacerbation of any complaint after treatment, and then reassure them that this is the normal progress of treatment. Most people understand the concept of things sometimes having to get worse before they get better. But you must emphasize that such episodes are always brief and should pass within a day or so. If they do not, other factors, apart from the Law of Cure, are involved.

An example of the Law of Cure in operation is that of a patient who had scarlet fever in childhood, which was accompanied by high fever, a hot rash and some secondary infections, such as earache. She was treated by antibiotics which hastened her recovery, but suppressed some of the symptoms. As her acupuncture treatment progressed, she re-experienced a sharp attack of earache for a day and her body developed a brief rash, signs that treatment had brought the suppressed symptoms to the surface to be expelled.

THE PATIENT'S ROLE IN TREATMENT

So far we have assumed that we as practitioners will be doing all the work. This is not appropriate if we want a balanced relationship with our patients. Patients need to understand that they are expected to contribute in many ways to the success of treatment. It is therefore important at the start of treatment to set out the terms under which we are prepared to treat patients. These can include the following conditions the patient must accept:

- Arriving on time
- Paying an agreed fee for each treatment where this is appropriate
- Paying if treatment is cancelled without notice or if the patient fails to arrive
- Contributing towards the success of treatment by willingly undertaking any lifestyle changes the practitioner suggests, such as taking more exercise, changing eating habits, eating more healthily
- Being truthful about alcohol, tobacco and drug consumption
- Not drinking alcohol for 24 hours before or after treatment
- Accepting the practitioner's judgement as to the frequency of treatment required
- Agreeing to accept the forms of treatment the practitioner selects (that is, needling whatever points are required, moxibustion on points)

CHAPTER 6

Acupuncture Points

Specific groups of points

When we insert a needle into an acupuncture point we are attempting in some way to affect the flow of energy along the meridians on which the selected acupuncture point lies. Many points are available to us, traditionally 365, but many more than these are known, and many points are rarely used. There are thus 365 or more access points to a patient's energy, and thus 365 or more different ways of approaching and helping the elements and their officials to which they relate. Acupuncture points are the means by which our treatment can help transform ill-health to health and despair to joy.

In practice, we use only a few of these points, those whose effectiveness tradition and practice have proved over time, and different traditions use less or more of some points than others. Each practitioner will develop their own repertoire of points for which they have a particular affinity, but some points form part of the standard repertoire for all practitioners. Each practitioner will add his/her own knowledge and experience of the points to the store of accumulated knowledge which has grown up over the millennia.

At the very heart of five element practice lies an understanding and use of what it calls the spirit of each individual point. Each point is seen as contributing a slightly different quality to the actions of the official to which it belongs. The power residing within each point therefore touches upon the deepest areas of human experience. And the practice of five element acupuncture is kind to its practitioners. It allows us to select the very simplest treatments and yet touch profound depths within our patients. The mere awareness of the profound nature of what we are doing adds depth to each simple treatment.

The point names we use in five element acupuncture are in English, and are those listed in J.R. Worsley's *The Meridians of Ch'i Energy: Point Reference Guide*.[*] One of the reasons for using English point names is that five element acupuncturists are encouraged to think of what we call the spirit of the point

---

[*] Worsley, J.R. (1979) *The Meridians of Ch'i Energy: Point Reference Guide.* Maryland: The Traditional Acupuncture Institute, Inc.

embedded in its name. Only profound Chinese scholars, such as Elisabeth Rochat de la Vallée, can get close to even a glimpse of the meaning hidden deep within the Chinese characters which form each point's name. I cannot do that, but I can hear J.R. Worsley guiding us through each point, infusing its name with some of the mystery inherent in the official to which it belongs and giving it a function for which it can be used. I am therefore happy to accept his listing of English point names as his particular take on the actions of these points. They represent my inheritance of a tradition.

The individual characteristic of a point is indicated to a greater or lesser extent in the name it has been given since acupuncture's earliest days, and about which there is much discussion. Some point names, such as IX 8 (Lu 8), Meridian Gutter, or XI 40 (St 40), Abundant Splendour, clearly indicate their function; others are more obscure. For these we have to call on a rich tradition which underlies our understanding of the functions of these points.

The point locations used are those set out in J.R. Worsley's *Traditional Chinese Acupuncture, Vol 1 Meridians and Points*.** There is much discussion about the location of certain points, such as IV 3 or IV 4 (Ki 3 or Ki 4), but such debates form part of the organic nature of acupuncture. I defy anybody to state categorically that a point is in one place rather than a few millimetres to the right or left. I suspect, but of course can never know, that the meridians do not run in the beautiful straight lines shown on our charts, but perfuse their energy over a wider area both below and around the meridian pathways. I am sure that it is therefore possible to summon energy to the needle both by needling in different ways (hence the many different needling techniques devised) and by needling at slightly different locations (hence the different locations devised). I think this is one of the reasons why different schools of acupuncture insist on different locations for their points, each no doubt for their own compelling reasons. Whatever the method of point location or of needling used, the essential thing here is whether we feel we have contacted a point and released or stimulated its energy, and that the intended result is achieved. How and where that contact is made will always remain a matter of debate.

SPECIFIC GROUPS OF POINTS
Command points
At the start of treatment, we use points which come mainly from the group we call command points. These address the officials in the most direct, and at

---

**   Worsley, J.R. (1975) *Traditional Chinese Acupuncture, Vol 1 Meridians and Points*. Tisbury: Element Books.

the same time the safest, way and put the officials under pressure to declare themselves in their true colours. They create a safe entrance to deeper work upon the officials. The command points form the bricks with which we work. Some of the cement we add to make the foundations more solid will come from other powerful points, such as those on Conception or Governor Vessels and specific Kidney or Bladder points, which we will discuss later.

Command points offer a profound and direct point of access to the elements themselves. This treatment alone will gradually bring about transformation. If we learn slowly to add to it some of the power other points can bring to what we are doing, we will speed up the action of the command points a little, that is all. We can address the guardian element in many ways, in the simple and effective words of the command points, or in the more complex sentences which other points can add to these words. But in the end, provided we address it with the full focus of our understanding and envelop our treatment in the warmth of our spirit, command points alone will bring transformation.

Command points lie between the fingertips and the elbow or between the toes and the knee, depending on the meridian involved. All have their own in-built safety mechanisms, and are therefore the safest points to use. They have a direct line of connection to each official, and form the bedrock of any treatment because they leave the patient in control of their own energy. Some treatments will consist only of needling command points. This is particularly true at the start of treatment, when each needle inserted is asking the question of the practitioner, 'Am I correctly addressing the needs of the guardian element?'

There are six groups of command point, as follows.

1. Source points
This is the most important group of all command points. They provide direct access to the officials, and are a way of gaining direct information about the guardian element's response to treatment. If used at the end of treatment they put the patient back in control of their own energy. They are the command points selected to complete the first treatment.

2. Element points
The largest group of command points is that of the element points, each meridian having element points which relate to each of the five elements. Element points add something of the quality of that particular element to the official concerned. The Metal element point on a Fire official will therefore add some of the quality and hardness of Metal to the Fire element. The

Earth element point on a Water official will add some of Earth's solidity and nurturing to the Water element.

The element points are spaced along the meridians in the following pattern:

- Yin meridians: All nail points on finger or toe are points which relate to the Wood element. The sequence of points which continues up to the elbow or knee then follows the Sheng cycle, finishing at the elbow or knee with Water points. All the source points on yin meridians are Earth points.

- Yang meridians: All nail points are points on finger or toe which relate to the Metal element. The sequence of points which continues up to the elbow or knee then follows the Sheng cycle, finishing at the elbow or knee with Earth points. The source points on yang meridians are not element points.

The other element points between nail and elbow/knee are spaced out at different intervals on different meridians, sometimes following on one from another and sometimes interspersed with non-command points (see below).

3. Horary/seasonal points

At a specific time of day and in a specific season, the element point of the official's element becomes a horary and/or seasonal point, and has the effect of clearing out debris from the official so that its true state of energy can be revealed. For example, III 66 (Bl 66) and IV 10 (Ki 10), both Water points, are the horary/seasonal points on their respective meridians. They are used at the officials' time according to the Chinese clock (15:00–17:00 and 17:00–19:00 respectively) or in their season, winter. Horary/seasonal points, especially when used in combination (that is, during the element's season as well as at their horary times) are the most powerful treatment at the command point level to be given a patient.

For a further discussion of these points see also Chapter 9.

4. Junction points

These connect the energy between the paired yin and yang officials within an element. They can be used to correct an imbalance between the two which a pulse reading will detect. To correct this, energy is drawn to the deficient official using its junction points. For example, if the pulses reveal that the Lung has less energy than the Large Intestine, a pulse reading known as a split pulse, the junction point on the Lung, IX 7 (Lu 7), is needled using tonification technique to draw energy from its stronger sister official. Split pulses between officials within an element are uncommon, since yin and yang officials will strive to share their energy between them, but they can occur, particularly if one or other official has been under a great deal of stress.

5. Tonification points

A tonification point is one that draws energy from mother to child element. For example V 9 and VI 3 (HP 9 and TH 3), both Wood points, are tonification points on their respective meridians. They draw energy from the mother element, Wood, to its child, Fire. A tonification needle technique is used with these points.

6. Sedation points

A sedation point is one that is used to push energy away from mother to child element, for example, XII 5 and XI 45 (Sp 5 and St 45), both Metal points, are sedation points on their respective meridians. They push energy away from the mother element, Earth, to its child, Metal. A sedation needling technique is used with these points.

Both tonification and sedation points are ways of transferring energy around the cycle of the elements. For further discussion of energy transfers see also Chapter 9. Command points can have several functions, to be used in one capacity or another as required. VII 38 (GB 38), for example, is a Fire and a sedation point on the Gall Bladder, I 7 (Ht 7) a source point, a sedation point and an Earth point on the Heart.

Non-command points

Finally, there are some points at command-point level which have no relationship to any element and no specific function, except for what they offer to their respective element in terms of what we call their spirit. These are called non-command points. X 7 (LI 7) and IV 5 (Ki 5) are two such points.

Associated Effect Points

Each official has a corresponding Associated Effect Point (AEP) (back shu point) on the Bladder meridian, which provides a direct channel of communication to the organ itself. This direct means of access makes these into very powerful points. AEPs are considered by some to be command points, but unlike those on the arm and leg, which have their own in-built safety factor, they have no such safety factor to control their effects, and they must therefore be used with care. In particular, they must only be used after any Aggressive Energy present has been drained, since it will otherwise be driven further inside as the AEPs are needled.

All AEPs lie on the Inner Bladder line on the back, but they do not affect the Bladder official when used. After using an AEP, a command point on the corresponding official should be used to tether the treatment and return control to the patient.

The AEPs of both yin and yang officials should be needled together, yang first, then yin. The only exception to this rule may be in the case of the Heart AEP, when it may not always be considered necessary to needle it in conjunction with the Small Intestine AEP, on the five element principle that we avoid needling the Heart where possible.

The AEPs are the following Bladder points:

- III 13 (Bl 13) Lung
- III 14 (Bl 14) Heart Protector
- III 15 (Bl 15) Heart
- III 18 (Bl 18) Liver
- III 19 (Bl 19) Gall Bladder
- III 20 (Bl 20) Spleen
- III 21 (Bl 21) Stomach
- III 22 (Bl 22) Three Heater
- III 23 (Bl 23) Kidney
- III 25 (Bl 25) Large Intestine
- III 27 (Bl 27) Small Intestine
- III 28 (Bl 28) Bladder

Windows of the Sky

A further group of points are those represented by the points called the Windows of the Sky. Their function is to act as connecting points to the world outside, opening our eyes to what lies beyond us. Often when we are out of balance we sink deep within ourselves, and lose our sense of what is going on around us and where we fit into the scheme of things. At some stage in treatment it is important for patients to re-establish this lost contact, and to move out beyond themselves and their own problems. These points are a way of doing this. They help patients find a perspective from which to view their own concerns. They provide an opening through which they can learn to see things as they are, which is the mark of balance.

Windows in a house are there to be shut as well as to let in the light, and if we are balanced we should be able to do both. Our good energy will help us decide when we have taken in too much so that we need to close our windows or when we need a little more light to see by, and open them. When we are out of balance the windows may remain tightly shut so that we remain locked in a dark, small room, as though in solitary confinement. We can be unable to see our way forward and become stuck in an emotion or a situation. Using these points will allow us to learn how to open and shut the windows to our soul appropriately.

These are very powerful points and not used lightly or early on in treatment. Energy has to be built up, so that a patient can deal with the influx of new light. It would be unwise to allow too much light to stream in when a person has been in the dark for a long time. As T.S. Eliot says in 'The Four Quartets', 'Mankind cannot bear too much reality.' We have to be cautious when using these points and ensure that the reality of their life which these points lay bare is not too painful for a patient to see.

Not all people need these points. Some patients are already very self-aware when they come for treatment. Yet others need these points quite frequently if they are going through phases of transition where it is important to let in enough light to enable them to see their way forward.

The Window chosen should be on the patient's element, and treatment should always be completed with command points on this element. The Metal element and Outer Fire are the only elements to have paired Windows on both their officials. These should be needled together, yang first, then yin.

Not every official has a Window, and it is interesting to see the distribution of the points amongst officials, as it tells us quite a lot about the functions of these officials. It is noticeable, for example, that the only official to have two Windows is the Small Intestine. This can be seen as fitting for an official which acts as the closest protector of the Heart, providing it with the additional vision it requires to ensure that it is able to guide the Heart wisely. It is also intriguing that there is no official Window listed for the Wood element, probably because Wood's close association with vision means that each Wood point in some way opens us up to the future and to what lies before us.

Windows of the Sky

Small Intestine	II 16 (SI 16)	Heavenly Window
	II 17 (SI 17)	Heavenly Appearance
Bladder	III 10 (Bl 10)	Heavenly Pillar
Heart Protector	V 1 (HP 1)	Heavenly Pond (for men)
	V 2 (HP 2)	Heavenly Spring (for women)
Three Heater	VI 16 (TH 16)	Heavenly Window
Lung	IX 3 (Lu 3)	Heavenly Palace
Large Intestine	X 18 (LI 18)	Support and Rush Out
Stomach	XI 9 (St 9)	People Welcome
Conception Vessel	CV 22	Heaven Rushing Out
Governor Vessel	GV 16	Wind Palace

CHAPTER 7

BLOCKS TO TREATMENT

Possession
Aggressive Energy
The Law of Husband-Wife
Entry-Exit blocks
Blocks caused by scars

The energy circling through the meridians can become blocked in different ways and for different reasons, preventing the elements from maintaining health as they should. These blocks can appear at different intervals, but all need to be cleared for treatment to progress as it should.

There are five major sources of blocked energy.

POSSESSION: The seven internal and external dragons
The protocol for diagnosing and treating possession harks back to a time when spirits were seen as ruling the world, and the forces of life, including health and ill-health, were personified as good or evil spirits. The deep imbalance of the spirit, which we would now diagnose as schizophrenia or psychosis, is here personified as possession by evil spirits, devils or demons. One picturesque phrase used by Paul Unschuld is 'the curse of the ancestor'.

In modern religious thought, possession by evil spirits is still very much an accepted condition, and there are procedures for exorcizing these evil spirits in many traditions, from Christianity to voodoo. This is confirmation, if it is needed, that a condition in which a person appears to be in the power of some force over which he/she has no control is accepted as existing. The term, possession, therefore remains with us here in the 21st century, although there is a strong case for removing the word from a five element acupuncturist's vocabulary precisely because of its archaic overtones, which bring with them a strong whiff of the supernatural.

There is nothing supernatural at all about possession in a patient. It forms part, instead, of a patient's natural defence mechanism which has come into play to protect him/her from deeper emotional damage. In severe cases, the patient may indeed feel as if they are in the grip of a force which controls them, but it is best seen as a loss of control over themselves, not a force imposing itself from outside.

An extreme example of possession is the schizophrenic or psychotic person. At a less extreme range, possession may be imperceptible to all but the most acute observer, showing itself only as slightly odd or abnormal behaviour. We feel that we can't quite reach the person, and when we approach them, we come up against a sense of blankness rather than the normal contact we establish when we meet people.

Treatment to clear possession is one of the most rewarding and effective forms of five element treatment. The practitioner summons the seven Internal or seven External Dragons to his/her aid to chase the devils away. In more modern terminology, the needling of the seven Dragon points acts as a form of re-connection, enabling the patient's spirit to emerge from behind its defensive screen. A sign that possession has cleared is the establishment of eye contact as the needles do their work, replacing the former blankness and detachment of spirit which characterizes this imbalance.

Why does possession occur?
For possession to take hold, a patient must have been subjected to some prolonged or extreme trauma which is so severe that our normal defence mechanisms can no longer cope. We protect ourselves from further pain by retreating into an inner world where we make ourselves safe. In some ways, possession can be seen as something akin to a state of extended shock, which can remain unperceived by others, except when it is extreme. Any major trauma or prolonged stress, such as drug, alcohol, sexual or physical abuse, can lead to possession. An overwhelming event, such as the sudden death of a parent in childhood, can also be a cause.

A possessed person is often one in whom the body and mind may function apparently normally, but the spirit retreats damaged behind a barrier. A person may therefore be able to hold down a job, whilst only the most sensitive observer will notice that anything is wrong. As the condition becomes more severe, however, the mind and body, too, will become impaired, until there is the total breakdown we recognize in a completely disturbed patient, where neither body nor soul work as they should. The patient will cease to function normally to a point where it is obvious to everybody that there is severe disturbance.

Those in the presence of possession often feel disorientated themselves, as though unsure of what exactly is going on. The patient's spirit has lost its bearings, and draws us with it into a world where the normal rules of behaviour gradually cease to exist. It may be difficult to follow what the patient is saying, as their speech reflects this disorder, and in extreme cases patients themselves will speak of being taken over by other forces. Often possessed people say things like, 'Something inside me made me do this…' One patient said, 'There are devils inside my head telling me what to do.'

How to detect possession

The only confirmation of the presence of possession is to look into a patient's eyes, and try to contact their spirit with your spirit. The eyes are the windows of the soul, and will reflect the presence or absence of a patient's spirit. The patient should be asked to look into one of your eyes, and you return the look, focusing also on that one eye, with the strength of your gaze attempting to establish contact with the patient's spirit. Where there is no possession, the patient will become uncomfortable under such a direct gaze, and blink or move slightly in response. In a possessed person there is no response at all, and you feel as if you are coming up against a blankness or emptiness.

With experience, we grow to recognize the presence or absence of the patient's spirit. It is not easy to detect at first, which is why all practitioners should practise by looking into each patient's eye as a part of each diagnosis.

Treatment of possession

Treatment is called releasing the seven dragons to fight the demons, and the points used are called Internal and External Dragons, known as IDs and EDs. In my own practice I have not found it at all easy to differentiate between these two forms of imbalance. A case of what could be regarded as an external cause of possession, such as prolonged exposure to abuse, may clear itself with treatment by IDs and something with a clearer internal cause, such as alcohol abuse, may require EDs to clear it.

Treatment always starts with IDs, and moves on to EDs only in the comparatively rare cases where the IDs are insufficient. In each case sedation is used first (the dragons pacifying the demons), then tonification (the dragons driving the demons out).

Seven needles are used for each set of dragons, and contact has to be made with each point in turn if treatment is to be successful. This is much like operating a combination lock in which each bolt has to fall in place before the combination releases the lock.

Possession treatment is always followed by testing for and clearing Aggressive Energy, even if this has been done before, since possession can mask its presence.

Procedure for IDs

- The pulses are checked and recorded. Often the clearing of possession will reveal itself in a pulse change.
- The following points are marked (7 points in all):
  - Master point in the depression just below CV 15 (about ½cm below)
  - XI 25 (St 25) (bilaterally)
  - XI 32 (St 32) (bilaterally)
  - XI 41 (St 41) (bilaterally)
- Needles are inserted in the following manner:
  - From top to bottom of the body (that is, master point below CV 15 first)
  - From right to left, with a hint of sedation
  - They are inserted straight, and should stand up firmly once inserted, confirming that contact has been made and is maintained. If the needle falls over, it should be inserted more deeply
- The patient is asked to feed back when he/she feels each point connect. If one needle does not contact its point, re-position it until it does. If all are not in place, the treatment will not work.
- When all needles have been inserted correctly, each point is sedated fully (180° anti-clockwise) in the order of insertion, that is, right then left, and the needles left in.
- They can be left in for up to 20 minutes, but can be removed before this in the order of insertion if possession has cleared. Usually it takes only a few minutes for possession to clear if all the needles are in the correct position. Eye contact should be checked at intervals to see whether normal eye-to-eye contact is now taking place.
- If possession has not cleared after 20 minutes, each point should be tonified strongly in the order of insertion but this time from left to right, and each needle removed in turn.

- A further check to see whether possession has cleared should be made.
  * If it has cleared, proceed to do an AE drain.
  * If it has not cleared, move on to do the EDs.

Procedure for EDs

- Repeat the same procedure as for IDs using the following points:
  * GV 20
  * III 11 (Bl 11) (bilaterally)
  * III 23 (Bl 23) (bilaterally)
  * III 61 (Bl 61) (bilaterally)

If you are sure that possession has not yet cleared by the end of the ID/ED procedure, do not proceed to do the AE drain, but finish the treatment with the source points of the patient's element. Ask the patient to come back so that you can repeat the whole procedure. It is unusual not to clear possession the first time, provided you are properly focused and are sure that you have contacted all the points, but there may be cases where possession is so entrenched that it requires one or two treatments to clear it.

If you think that you will need to do this treatment, make sure you have left enough time in your diary for this long procedure (IDs, followed by AE drain, followed by the source points of the guardian element). Since possession has usually been there for some time, if not for many years, it will not matter if you wait to do this treatment until the next time the patient comes. The important thing is not to be in a hurry and always to allow yourself plenty of time.

AGGRESSIVE ENERGY

Aggressive Energy (AE) forms part of the five element understanding of the concept of polluted energy within a person. It can be regarded as another name for negative energy or perverse qi. The term is thought to have first been used in the 1960s by Jacques Lavier, who was one of the teachers of J.R. Worsley. According to Lavier, there are two ways of draining this negative energy:

- Through the Associated Effect Points (back shu points)
- Through the five element command points

Only the first method is now used in five element acupuncture. Other traditions, such as modern TCM, use the second method for eliminating negative energy.

In five element acupuncture the presence of Aggressive Energy is regarded as forming one of the major blocks to treatment, and has to be cleared before treatment can start to be effective. The diagnosis as to whether there is AE, and the treatment to eliminate it if it is there, are carried out at one and the same time, using the Associated Effect Points (AEPs) (back shu points) of the yin organs.

Aggressive Energy occurs as the result of continuous stress or trauma hammering away at an element until its defences weaken. It is called Aggressive Energy, because as the element weakens, its energy, instead of being the life-giving force it is in health, becomes destructive and turns in upon the patient. Once this happens, the element tries to get rid of its destructive energy by passing it on, and it does this as far as possible by protecting its child according to the Law of Mother-Child. It therefore pushes AE away from its child across the cycle to its grandchild using the Ke cycle of energy. When AE is present, the Ke cycle becomes a destructive cycle. In all other circumstances, it is a cycle of control.

If Fire is in trouble, for example, it will pass its polluted energy, not to Earth, its child, but to Metal, its grandchild. If the AE received by Metal is too powerful for it to resist, Metal, in turn, will be unable to deal with it and will pass it on to its grandchild, Wood, and so on.

In acupuncture terms, death is the result of AE passing round the Ke cycle in such a destructive manner that each element in turn becomes polluted, and there is no longer sufficient healthy energy to sustain life. For example, AE can pass across the Ke cycle from Wood to Earth, and then from Earth to Water and from Water to Fire, until all the elements succumb. In Western medicine, the equivalent is the kidney failure (Water element in distress) which precedes cardiac failure (Fire element in distress).

AE is found only on the yin organs. The yang organs, being hollow and passing energy directly to the outside, are able to disperse AE outwards.

Causes of AE

- Long-term stress, weakening the elements
- Severe trauma of any kind, including radiotherapy, chemotherapy or sudden or prolonged shock

Why AE might recur

The appearance of AE is a sign that the body is under attack. If this attack continues, AE may recur unless a patient's element is strengthened by treatment to withstand further stress. This is done by treating it at a sufficiently deep level and sufficiently often. If a patient is not improving or is getting worse, you should always check for AE again, just to make sure you eliminated it to start with. If AE is there, you should question either whether you did not tap for it correctly in the first place, or whether it has recurred because your treatment is not focused upon the right element or because the patient is continuing to be under great stress.

Some tips to help you suspect there might be AE

- Patient showing extreme emotional instability which indicates that different elements are under stress
- Tendency for the patient to burst into tears
- Pain around the chest and upper back
- Tightness around the area of the AEPs, particularly at the level of the Lung, Heart Protector and Heart
- Red striations across the back at the level of these AEPs
- White indentation around a needle when it is inserted as though it is being sucked into the skin. Red will appear around the needle very soon afterwards

Order of treatment for AE drain

AE is the first treatment to be carried out on every patient, except in the case of possession, where it is drained after possession has cleared. If AE is not drained, any treatment carried out whilst it is present will be ineffective, and may make a patient feel worse. Needling the AEPs at their correct needle insertion depth if there is AE can be very dangerous, as the needling will drive the AE deeper into the body and soul of the patient.

Procedure for diagnosing and draining AE

Needles are placed very shallowly in the skin. They should not be inserted so deeply that they protrude at right angles from the body, but should always lie at an angle of no more than 45° from the body. This is the only treatment in which needles are placed in this way. The intention is to avoid needling the point itself at its correct depth, but to open up a channel to the surface through which AE can escape from the body. Needling in this way makes it possible to drain any AE that is present without running the risk of pushing the AE further in.

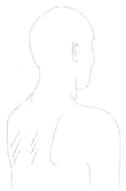

Needles are inserted bilaterally at each of the AEPs of the yin organs which are situated along the Inner Bladder line, as follows:

- AEP of Lung III 13 (Bl 13)
- AEP of Heart Protector III 14 (Bl 14)
- (AEP of Heart III 15 (Bl 15))
- AEP of Liver III 18 (Bl 18)
- AEP of Spleen III 20 (Bl 20)
- AEP of Kidney III 23 (Bl 23)

Needles are not inserted into the AEP of the Heart until AE has been confirmed on the Heart Protector needles. This is in accordance with the five element principle of avoiding needling the Heart wherever possible. When inserting the needles into the AEP of the Heart, particular care must be taken to ensure that they are not inserted too deeply. If AE has reached the Heart, too deep an insertion could force it deeper inside, which would be extremely dangerous.

Once the needles are inserted into all the AEPs, wait for 5–10 minutes to see whether red circular marks (erythema) develop around any of them. To ensure that the red marks are not merely caused by sensitivity to needles, extra needles (called dummy needles) are inserted close to the AEPs, but not at actual points. If these needles cause red markings to appear, you should wait until the erythema around the dummy needles dies down before deciding whether AE is present on the AEP needles.

AE can appear as faint or angry red markings from 0.5–2cm across around the AEP needles. If AE appears on an AEP on one side of the body but not on the other side, the needle on that side should be moved slightly in case it is not correctly placed. It is rare for AE to be present on one side only.

The needles must be left in until the erythema around them disappears. This may take from 20 minutes to 2 hours or more. If possible, you should give yourself enough time to ensure that all AE can be drained at one acupuncture session. It is therefore advisable to allow 2 hours for the first treatment. If another patient is waiting, and you have insufficient time to drain all the AE from the body, simply remove the needles without sealing the holes, and ask the patient to come back as soon as possible, completing the treatment with the source points of the patient's element.

Even though AE may still appear to be present when the patient leaves, it can continue to drain from the body even after the needles have been removed, so that there may be no sign of any AE when a patient returns. You must still, however, re-tap for AE at the next session to ensure that all has gone.

You can visualize the needles as protective lightning rods drawing negative energy away from the body.

How do you know when to remove the needles?

- A slight pinkish colouring around the needles may remain even after all AE has been drained. If it doesn't fade any further after 10–15 minutes, it may just be the skin's reaction to having a needle there. This means that AE has gone and you can safely remove the needles.

- There may be some erythema due to the needles, particularly on the AEPs of the Kidney, even when there is no AE there. Again, if the pink doesn't fade with time, it means there is no AE.

- If in doubt, leave the needles in a little longer. With practice you get to know what is AE and what isn't, and when it's still there and when it isn't.

Some useful tips

- You must always re-tap for AE after doing possession treatment. Possession will mask the presence of AE.

- If in doubt about where the AEPs are (and some backs are very difficult), palpate from the top to the bottom of the back and again from bottom to top to help you count the intervertebral spaces. With a very difficult back, where you are unsure of the numbering of the vertebrae, insert needles at the level of all the AEPs to make sure. Backs can be very crumpled or distorted, and it can be very difficult to feel exactly where the spaces are, so use every bit of help you can. The object is to drain AE, not to carry out an exercise in perfect point location.

- The recurrence of AE is a good warning sign not to be complacent. It may mean that we are not addressing some problem, either in our treatment (that is, the wrong element), or some lifestyle problem (excessive drinking, drug abuse or an abusive relationship, for example).

Some examples of AE from practice

- A patient had been given a high dose of radiotherapy for bone cancer which had spread throughout the body. Where she had had radiotherapy her back was burnt-looking, bright red and extremely sensitive to the touch. The AE drain caused the burnt colour to disappear from the body, leaving the back a healthy pink, and the patient freer from pain than she had been for a long time.

- A patient came for treatment suffering from extreme breathlessness and stabbing chest pains. All this disappeared after the AE drain.

- Another patient had severe back pain. This, too, disappeared after the AE drain.

THE LAW OF HUSBAND-WIFE

This law states that the sum total of energy of the left-hand pulses should be somewhat stronger in quality than the sum total of the pulses on the right-hand side. The pulses of the left side are called the husband's and those of the right side the wife's.

In a traditional society, the husband was seen as taking on the qualities of leadership in the outside world, and the wife those of leadership in the domestic world. Everybody has a husband and wife aspect inside themselves, their yang and yin aspects. Within man or woman, the husband aspect, which houses the Supreme Controller, the Heart, represented by the left-hand pulses, should be slightly stronger in quality and more in control, than the wife aspect, represented by the right-hand pulses. If the Heart loses control, life will be threatened.

A Husband-Wife (H/W) imbalance is characterized by a sense of resignation in the patient, and is revealed in the pulse picture by all the left-hand pulses showing serious depletion, whilst those of the right side pound with accumulated energy. Patients will often confirm the pulse reading by saying things like, 'I can't go on', 'I want to give up', 'I don't see any point in living.'

The imbalance is caused by trauma of some kind, which places considerable strain upon all the officials, particularly that arising from conflict or unhappiness in a relationship (the Heart unable to maintain control). For example, a man or woman may feel that he/she is being victimized in his/her relationship (wife side taking over more control than it should), or that more is demanded of him/her than he/she wishes to give (the husband side having to take more control than he/she wants).

It is important to remember that the difference between the two sets of pulses may not show itself as + pulses on the wife's side and -2 pulses on the husband's, but as a relative difference in pulse quality. The most significant pointer to a H/W imbalance is always a severe depletion in the Heart and Small Intestine pulses, as they struggle to survive. Another indicator will be the surprising strength in all the right-hand pulses given the patient's appearance of resignation and despair.

Treatment of a H/W imbalance

Treatment is very specific:

- Take from the wife and give to the husband: To do this, energy is drawn from all the officials on the wife's side to all those on the husband's side using energy transfers (see Chapter 9).

Correcting a H/W is essentially a very simple treatment with a profound and life-saving effect. If it is left uncorrected, the stress upon the Supreme Controller may be too great for it to bear, and it will go under, leading eventually to death. H/W must be treated immediately once diagnosed as it is considered life-threatening if left untreated.

Treatment procedure (moxa is not used for this procedure)

- Tonify III 67, IV 7 (Bl 67, Ki 7): Water (husband's side) is tonified by drawing energy from Metal (wife's side).
- Tonify IV 3 (Ki 3): Energy is transferred across the Ke cycle from the wife's side (Earth) to the husband's (Water).
- Tonify VIII 4 (Liv 4): Energy is transferred across the Ke cycle from the wife's side (Metal) to the husband's (Wood).

The treatment of the imbalance is completed by reinforcing the Supreme Controller, the Heart, and putting it back in control:

- Tonify II 4, I 7 (SI 4, Ht 7): Tonification of Heart and Small Intestine source points.
- Finally, the source points of the patient's element are tonified (with moxa if appropriate) to return control to the patient's guardian element.

The presence of a H/W imbalance is a sign of great stress upon the Heart. The patient should therefore be asked to come back for a further treatment within a few days to make sure that the imbalance has cleared. If it has not, the procedure is repeated until the H/W has been corrected.

ENTRY-EXIT BLOCKS

Energy flows in a circle from official to official and back again in a circle of energy called the Wei level. This is a defensive cycle of energy and lies at a more superficial level than the Sheng and the Ke cycles which flow from element to element. At the Wei level of circulation, the Heart passes energy to the Small Intestine which passes energy to the Bladder and so on around the circle of 12 officials in the numerical order used in five element acupuncture to indicate the officials (that is, from I to XII and back to I again).

The energy flowing at this level can become blocked between the end of one official and the beginning of the next. If it does, the energy is held back in one meridian, and not allowed to pass through to the next, as it should. This is called an Entry-Exit (E/E) block. A block of this kind can be diagnosed from the pulses. It can also appear as some form of imbalance in colour, sound, smell or emotion, or as a physical symptom around the area of the block.

There can also be an E/E block between the Conception and Governor Vessels, known as a CV/GV block. This is the most serious block of all E/E blocks, as it prevents these two major sources of energy from feeding the 12 officials. A block of this kind will show itself as great deficiency on all the pulses (-2 or lower on all 12), and appear as severe exhaustion. The patient will remain stubbornly resistant to treatment until the CV/GV block is cleared.

Blocks occur mainly between the end of one element and the start of the next, that is, the end of Wood and the start of Metal. It is rare for there to be a block within an element, for example between the Gall Bladder and the Liver, since the yin and yang officials will try to share their energy between them. It does, however, sometimes occur, and is known as a split pulse. This is treated by tonifying the junction point of the deficient official to equalize the energy between the two.

If there is an E/E block between Wood and Metal, a reading of the patient's pulses will show that the Liver and Gall Bladder (VIII and VII) have a relative excess of energy, and Metal officials, Lung and Large Intestine (IX and X), the next along the Wei cycle, have a relatively deficient amount of energy. It is as though the Liver is blocked at its exit point, VIII 14 (Liv 14), and is unable to pass its energy on to the Lung through its entry point, IX 1 (Lu 1). We call this an VIII/IX block. The pulse picture will show the Liver and Gall Bladder pulses as appearing full and tight, and the Lung and Large Intestine pulses as appearing empty. There may also be sensory changes indicating this relative imbalance, such as irrational anger, tight chest pains or a white colour (the Lung or Liver showing distress).

When E/E blocks occur

E/E blocks often occur a few weeks into treatment, although they may be there from the start. If they occur after a few treatments, they are a sign that energy at the deep level is improving and things are moving outwards towards the surface. Because they can cause symptoms which are temporarily unpleasant, it is helpful to reassure patients that they are a sign of improvement, rather than something to be concerned about.

The major block, the CV/GV block, is of another order, however, acting as a dam on all the energy flowing throughout the meridian system, and thus causing great depletion of energy in all the officials. The possibility of this block should be considered in all illnesses accompanied by severe and sustained lack of energy, such as multiple sclerosis and ME, where there is a gradual breakdown in the functioning of all the officials. It is also frequently found after surgery in childbirth, and accounts for the difficulties patients often experience when recovering from a Caesarian operation, or finding themselves unable to conceive.

Persistent E/E blocks, indicating that energy is only trickling through from one official to the next, may well be at the root of all manner of illnesses. It is likely, for instance, that Kidney-Heart Protector (IV/V) or Spleen-Heart (XII/I) blocks in women could either cause or, at the very least, exacerbate, the spread of breast cysts, since the good energy that would usually be flowing around the breast is now no longer flowing as it should.

If a patient comes to you with a history of breast problems, it is therefore important always to consider doing these blocks as a preventive measure, even if you are unsure that they are there from your pulse reading. The same is true of any long-term persistent pain in a specific area. It does no harm whatsoever to treat an E/E block if it is not there. This is like trying to open a gate which is already open. It is far worse to overlook a block which is there, since this pushes treatment up against a barred gate again and again.

There is a natural tendency for practitioners to be reluctant to diagnose and treat a CV/GV block, because of the location of CV 1. It is therefore important to be aware that we may be unconsciously convincing ourselves that the pulses are higher to avoid doing the treatment. It occurs surprisingly frequently, and the effects of clearing it are striking.

Once you decide there is an E/E block, it should be cleared straightaway, otherwise it will stop treatment from working. The blocks other than those between CV and GV do not always express themselves as a large difference between the two officials, but by a difference in quality, a tightness or hardness in the pulse of the exit official and a corresponding lack of energy in that of the adjacent official. CV/GV blocks prevent any improvement in the patient. Other blocks have less drastic effects, but can often have some side effects which may be unpleasant but brief.

Except in the case of a CV/GV block, the presence of an E/E block is a sign of energy hindered from moving round the Wei cycle. Always reassure patients, and yourself, that this is usually a good sign that energy is at last moving strongly through furred-up pathways unused to this amount of good energy flowing through them.

Treatment for all blocks except CV/GV

Treatment is simple, and very effective:

- Tonify the exit point of the excess official on both sides, yang first, then yin.

- Tonify the entry point of the deficient official on both sides, yang first, then yin.

In our example, we would tonify Liver's exit point, VIII 14 (Liv 14), to release the energy which has built up at the end of the Liver official. We would then tonify Lung's entry point, IX 1 (Lu 1), to draw this released energy towards the Lung.

Moxa is not used when clearing an Entry-Exit block. We are not trying to warm the points, but release their pent-up energy.

Treatment for a CV/GV block

- Tonify CV 1 and CV 24.
- Tonify GV 28 and GV 1.

CHAPTER 7: BLOCKS TO TREATMENT

Because of the location of CV 1 and GV 1, it is important that the patient is offered the choice of having a practitioner of their own sex needling these points. If the patient prefers to have their own practitioner of a different sex, then an observer of the same sex as the patient must always be present.

List of E/E points

The entry point is always the first point on each meridian, except in the case of the Large Intestine, where it is X 4 (LI 4). On the Heart Protector, V 2 (HP 2) acts as the entry point for women as it is forbidden on women to needle V 1 (HP 1), next to the nipple. The exit points differ from meridian to meridian.

	Entry	**Exit**
Heart	1	9
Small Intestine	1	19
Bladder	1	67
Kidney	1	22
Heart Protector	1 (2 for women)	8
Three Heater	1	22
Gall Bladder	1	41
Liver	1	14
Lung	1	7
Large Intestine	4	20
Stomach	1	42
Spleen	1	21
CV	1	24
GV	1	28

BLOCKS CAUSED BY SCARS

The scar tissue which forms after surgery or when we injure ourselves may block the flow of energy through the meridians at the site of the scarring. Energy will usually seek another route around or through the scar, but where there is severe, deep scarring this may be difficult. If a patient's treatment appears to have hit an impasse, it may be because energy is not flowing through the scar site as smoothly as elsewhere.

This is often the case if somebody has had major surgery, such as a hysterectomy or Caesarian operation, where there are scars cutting through the CV line and across other meridians.

Treatment

Treatment is simple.

- Points are needled using the tonification technique immediately below and above the scar, in the direction of the energy flow along the meridian. For example, if there is scarring on the leg across the Liver meridian between VIII 5 and VIII 6 (Liv 5 and 6), these two points are needled in the order of the flow of energy – VIII 5 (Liv 5) first, followed by VIII 6 (Liv 6). If there is scarring on the Bladder meridian between III 58 and 59 (Bl 58 and 59), III 58 (Bl 58) is needled first, followed by III 59 (Bl 59).

- Tonification is usually sufficient, but if this does not achieve the desired effect, the first point, VIII 5 (Liv 5) or III 58 (Bl 58), can be sedated, the needle left in, then VIII 6 (Liv 6) or III 59 (Bl 59) tonified to draw energy through and across the scar.

- If the scar lies across several meridians, the pulse picture should be used as a guide, and treatment should be directed at the officials showing greater distress. For example, if the scar lies across the Lung and the Heart Protector meridians on the hand, and only the Heart Protector pulses fail to improve with treatment, points above and below the scar on Heart Protector should be needled.

- In the case of surgery at the level of CV 2 (very common with Caesarians), CV 1 and CV 3 should be needled.

CHAPTER 8

Treatment Techniques

Needling techniques
Moxibustion techniques

The two treatment techniques in five element acupuncture which relate to the stimulation of acupuncture points are moxibustion and needling.

The use of herbs, as in other branches of acupuncture, is not a mainstream five element addition to treatment. In its emphasis upon complex refinements of the interrelationships of the elements and officials one to another, five element acupuncture does not on the whole lend itself to the application of herbs. Some acupuncturists have developed methods of categorizing some herbs according to elements, but the relationship of individual herbs to a corresponding element in the detail required for five element practice has not yet been studied sufficiently to make this part of everyday five element protocol.

At a less physical level, we must not forget the most profound treatment technique of all, if it can indeed be called by that name, which is the practitioner's relationship to the patient. Here we have to develop methods of treating our patients which call upon our ability to create an environment in which the patient feels safe and at ease both physically and emotionally. To do this, we also use certain physical skills, predominantly those of touch. Our hands can become instruments of profound healing if we learn how to make them conduits of our spirit so that in touching we offer our patients spiritual comfort. They can help us to convey a range of signals which bring reassurance and understanding to our patients. Our ability to use our hands in this way is a treatment technique at a profound level, by our skill enabling us to bridge the gap between one human being and another. The treatments we offer move to a deeper level if we add appropriate touch to the physical actions involved in needling and moxibustion.

NEEDLING TECHNIQUES

The needling technique used is based on that transmitted to J.R. Worsley through various teachers and is shared by Japanese schools of acupuncture. Its characteristic is that the practitioner as well as the patient must feel the sensation of contact with the point ('feeling the qi'). Another characteristic is the speed of needling when employing tonification technique, in which the needle is given a 180° turn in a clockwise direction and removed immediately contact is made with the point.

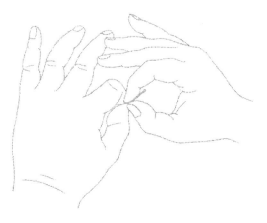

The sedation (dispersal) technique used in five element acupuncture is more akin to that used by other branches of acupuncture. The needle is left in the point for up to 20 minutes to disperse the energy. Sedation is used much less frequently since much of the need to disperse energy has been removed by the draining of Aggressive Energy, where each of the yin organs is encouraged to get rid of any excess energy from the body.

The act of needling forms as much a part of the relationship between practitioner and patient as the emotional rapport which five element acupuncturists feel must be established for treatment to be effective. As the practitioner needles the point, he/she is conscious of the connection to the patient which is being established through the needle, not only through the body but with the mind and spirit. This provides an explanation for the fact that students may be needling at the right location, needle depth and angle, and yet not contact the point, because they have not yet learned how to establish this essential connection.

The delicacy of touch used in Japanese needling also forms part of five element needling technique. The more skilful the needling technique, the less the patient will feel, although patients are more sensitive to the needling of particular points at different times, and there are many points which are always very sensitive.

CHAPTER 8: TREATMENT TECHNIQUES

Needling methods

There are five different methods of needling in the five element repertoire:

- Tonification
- Sedation
- Needling to transfer energy from element to element
- Needling to drain Aggressive Energy
- Needling to clear possession (Internal and External Dragons)

Tonification technique

Tonification is used when the pulse reading indicates that the energy of the element to be treated requires stimulating.

- The points are needled first on the left and then on the right.
- The needle is inserted at an angle of from 10–25° from the perpendicular in the direction of the flow of the meridian's energy.
- The needle is rotated 180° in a clockwise direction, and removed immediately contact is established.
- If contact is not immediately established, the needle angle or position should be changed slightly until contact is made. After removal of the needle the point is sealed immediately with the finger using sterile cotton wool.

Sedation technique

Sedation is used when the pulse reading indicates that the energy of the element to be treated requires dispersal.

- The points are needled first on the right and then on the left.
- The needle is inserted at an angle of from 10–25° from the perpendicular against the direction of flow of the meridian's energy.
- The needle is rotated 180° in an anti-clockwise direction and left in the point until the pulse reading indicates that sufficient energy has dispersed.
- The needle is then removed without further rotation, and the point is not sealed.

Needling to transfer energy from element to element
Here the needles are used to draw energy from one element to another. A specific technique is used (see Chapter 9).

Needling to drain Aggressive Energy
Here contact is not made with the meridian itself, but a pathway to the surface of the skin is created through which the Aggressive Energy in the meridians is drawn towards the surface and out of the body (see Chapter 7).

Needling to clear possession (Internal and External Dragons)
The needles are inserted according to the procedure outlined in Chapter 7.

MOXIBUSTION TECHNIQUES
The moxibustion technique used is based on that transmitted to J.R. Worsley through various teachers, one of the routes of transmission being from Japan. Different branches of acupuncture use different types of moxa, different sizes of moxa cones and different forms of moxibustion. Moxa can be applied on the needle, on a bed of salt or ginger, direct to the skin and in other ways. Its aim is always to warm the body, and specifically to warm the acupuncture point over which it is placed.

The technique used is to apply small, rice-sized cones of moxa punk to the acupuncture point, and light the cone with a taper. Once heated, the cone is allowed to burn down until the patient feels the heat, when it is removed, and a further cone applied. The cone should be removed before it touches the skin, but it may leave a slight brown mark. This is why moxa is not used in exposed areas of the body, such as the face.

The aim of moxibustion is to prepare the point for needling by warming it in advance so that the needle itself feels warm to the patient as it is inserted into the point. The application of heat to a point before needling is seen as enhancing the point's efficacy. Heat is regarded as warming not only the body but also the spirit, and prepares the point to welcome the needle.

The fact that a patient may appear to be flushed and have hot skin is not a contraindication to applying moxa, as it is in other traditions. It is also possible for people to feel warm to the touch and yet to feel cold inside. However warm the body, therefore, moxa will be applied to the points if it is felt that the patient's spirit can benefit from the warmth moxibustion brings to the point. It is therefore customary to apply moxa to all points unless this is contraindicated.

Moxa stimulates the point and is therefore only used before tonifying a point, if the energy requires stimulating. It is not used before sedation, if the energy requires dispersing.

Size and number of moxa cones

The size of the moxa cone is determined by the need for the point to be warmed and then to retain heat for a sufficiently long time so that each new application adds heat. If the cone is too large, it takes too long to heat the point, and this allows the point to cool down between applications. If the cone is too small, it heats the point too rapidly and the point does not retain the heat.

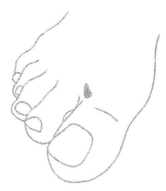

The moxa punk used for this type of moxibustion is Chinese, which burns more slowly than Japanese moxa, and is regarded as providing the correct amount of heat for repeated applications.

The minimum and maximum number of cones is specified for each point. The numbers range from 2–50, with an average number of 3–5. The minimum number of moxa cones is used to start with. This number can increase gradually to the maximum recommended number if the point is repeated at a future date and if the practitioner feels that the patient will benefit from more warmth.

How to apply moxa cones

The moxa is rolled firmly between the fingers to form a cone the size of a grain of rice. The patient's skin is slightly moistened for the first application to enable the cone to remain in place. The cone is lit with a taper, and left to smoulder down until the patient feels the heat. It is then removed and extinguished by pressing the thumb and little finger firmly on it. These are the two fingers traditionally used, as the slight scarring to the practitioner's fingers which results from frequent moxa applications would impair the sensitivity of the three middle, pulse-taking fingers.

The residual moxa left on the point on removal will usually be enough for subsequent cones to be applied without further moistening of the skin. Cones can be applied in this way at any angle of the body, for example to the back with the patient sitting up.

If the points on the left and right sides of the meridian are to be needled on opposite sides of the treatment couch, moxa should be applied to the point on one side of the body, and the point needled immediately whilst it is still warm. The procedure is then repeated on the other side.

If the points on the left and right side lie close enough to be needled without moving round the couch, as for example the Associated Effect Points or the source points of Stomach and Spleen, an experienced acupuncturist will stagger the moxa applications in such a way that a cone on the left point can be heated as one on the right is removed. Both points will then remain warm enough to be needled consecutively.

It requires some practice to gain sufficient dexterity to do this; a newly qualified acupuncturist will be better advised to apply cones to one side at a time.

Moxa cones applied to CV 8

There is one exception to the size of the cones. When moxa is applied to CV 8, on the umbilicus, it is placed on a bed of salt which fills the umbilicus to the level of the surrounding skin. The cones therefore have to be sufficiently large to heat the salt beneath them. The size of the cone depends upon the width and depth of the umbilicus. A narrow and shallow umbilicus will require less salt and therefore smaller moxa cones to heat it, whilst a wide and deep umbilicus will require correspondingly more salt and larger moxa cones. The cones can be from 1–2cm in height, and should be wide enough at the base to cover the umbilicus.

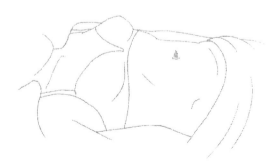

Unlike the normal application, where the burnt moxa cone is replaced immediately by another cone, the salt must be allowed to cool for a minute before the next cone is placed on it. If this is not done, the umbilicus will become too hot and the delicate skin inside can become burnt. Care must also be taken to ensure that there remains a sufficiently large bed of salt on which to place each successive cone so that burning moxa can at no point touch the skin.

Contraindications to moxibustion

- If the patient's BP is high, or there is a diastolic/systolic differential of more than 40
- If moxibustion is forbidden for that point

CHAPTER 9

Treatment Protocols

The Law of Mother-Child and Sheng and Ke cycles
Energy transfers
Seasonal and daily treatment cycles

THE LAW OF MOTHER-CHILD AND SHENG AND KE CYCLES

Underlying much of five element treatment is one of the fundamental laws of acupuncture, the law of Mother-Child. According to this, each element is regarded as the child of the preceding element and the mother of the following element along the cycle which flows clockwise from Wood, Fire, Earth, Metal to Water and back to Wood again.

Energy passes from element to element in this way, creating the cycle of energy called the Sheng cycle. Energy also passes from one yang official on one element to the yang official on the next element, and from one yin official to the next, that is, from Large Intestine to Bladder and from Lung to Kidney. In the case of the Fire element, the Gall Bladder will pass its energy to both the Small Intestine and the Three Heater, the Liver to the Heart and the Heart Protector.

Energy can also be passed across the cycle, again in a clockwise direction, so that a mother element can pass her energy to her grandchild. This is called the Ke cycle of energy. Energy passed across the cycle in this way passes only from one yin official to another. Junction points can be used to connect the energy of the yin and yang officials if this is required.

The Ke cycle is a cycle of control, and unlike the Sheng cycle can become destructive, as it does in the case of Aggressive Energy.

ENERGY TRANSFERS

The practice of transferring energy using one or other or both of the Sheng and Ke cycles is a characteristic of five element acupuncture, and does not appear to be used by other schools of acupuncture. It appears first in teachings by the French acupuncturists, Soulié de Morant and Lavier, and was apparently part of the teaching by Niboyet transmitted to J.R. Worsley in 1963.

The aim of any transfer of energy is to balance the relative energy shared between the elements and officials so that none retains more energy than another. This way of redistributing energy helps to resolve tension between all the officials, and is an amazingly simple and effective way of restoring harmony. Transferring energy in this way is therefore one of the most powerful and effective forms of treatment since it benefits all the elements by reducing disparities between them.

We use energy transfers to support the guardian element by transferring to it relatively excess energy from elsewhere. The energy distributes itself most generously when this element is given the treatment to enable it to re-establish its dominant position in the hierarchy of the elements. If the guardian element is struggling, the other elements are called upon to help it, and will show their relief once it is back in control.

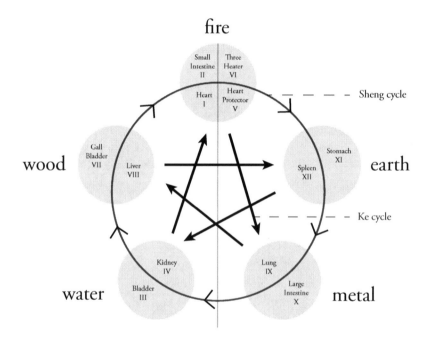

Transfers using the Sheng cycle

- Tonification: Drawing energy to a relatively deficient element/official (using tonification needling technique). Here energy is transferred from mother element to child element, using the connection of yin to yin official and yang to yang official. If the guardian element is deficient, we use the yin and yang tonification points on its mother element to do this transfer. If the guardian element has excess energy, we use its yin and yang sedation points to push energy away from it towards its child.

- Sedation: Dispersing energy from a relatively excess element/official (using the sedation needling technique). Here energy is drawn to or transferred from the element/officials in a mother-child relationship to one another.

Example 1
Tonification of Earth:
XI 41 (St 41), XII 2 (Sp 2)
(Fire points of Stomach and Spleen)

Example 2
Sedation of Earth:
XI 45 (St 45), XII 5 (Sp 5)
(Metal points of Stomach and Spleen)

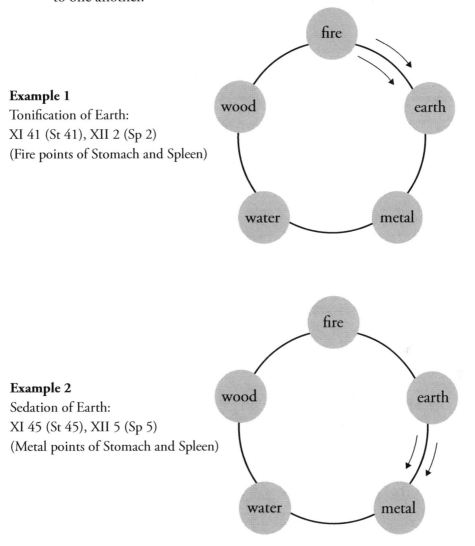

Transfers using the Ke cycle

These can only be used to draw energy to the guardian element, not away from it. There are two forms of transfer here, a simple and a more complex form.

- Simple transfer: This transfer is across the Ke cycle from the yin official of a grandmother element to the yin official of its grandchild.

Example 1
Transfer from Wood to Earth:
XII 1 (Sp 1)
(Wood point of Spleen)

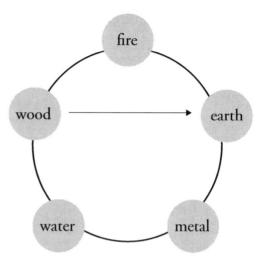

- More complex transfers: Here energy is passed further along the cycle, that is, from great-grandmother to great-grandchild element, and an intermediary element is used as carrier element, according to the following procedure.

Example 2
Transfer from Earth to Wood:

Needle 1
VIII 4 (Liv 4)
(Metal point of Liver)

Needle 2 (carrier needle)
IX 9 (Lu 9)
(Earth point of Lung)

(An alternative route from Earth to Water to Wood can also be used)

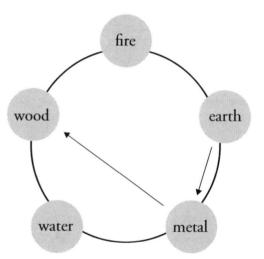

Procedure for transferring energy

- The shortest transfer route is chosen and the least number of needles used.

- A route through the Heart official is avoided where possible, since the Heart is considered a sacred organ following the Japanese tradition.
- The route always follows the cycle of generation of the elements (that is, clockwise).
- If the route passes through another element or official, this element or official acts as a carrier, and does not take away energy as energy passes through it.

Needling procedure

- In all cases, the needle is inserted first on the left, then on the right.
- Needles are inserted into the deficient element first with a hint of tonification, and are left in place.
- Needles are inserted into any carrier official with a hint of tonification and left in place.
- No needles are inserted into the excess element from which energy is being drawn.
- Finally, the needles in the deficient element are tonified fully, and removed immediately.
- The remaining needles in the carrier official(s) are removed without further tonification.
- If necessary, energy can then be transferred from the yin official to its paired yang official using the junction point between them, but this is rarely necessary, since the two officials usually balance their energy out between them.

Theoretically, it is possible to transfer energy from any official or element in the five element cycle to any other, always following the direction of the flow of energy, but in practice some transfers are more frequently done than others, since certain elements tend to have more energy than others. For example, the Wood and Earth officials are usually relatively stronger than the Water and Heart Protector/Three Heater officials, which are called upon to provide our reserves of energy.

The following are therefore the most common transfers used:

- To Outer Fire: V 3 (HP 3), IV 3 (Ki 3) (from Earth to Fire)

- To Wood: VIII 4 (Li 4) (from Metal to Wood); IX 9 (Lu 9), VIII 4 (Li 4) (from Earth to Wood)
- To Earth: XII 1 (Sp 1) (from Wood to Earth)

Transfers involving the Fire element

For the purposes of energy transfers, the inner and outer aspects of the Fire element are considered to be two elements. Energy cannot pass from one side of Fire directly to the other. If the Small Intestine is asked to feed the Three Heater, energy must therefore be transferred right round the cycle, until it is drawn to the other side of Fire. In practice, this is never done, but it is theoretically possible.

Energy transfers from one official within an element to its yin or yang sister official within the same element

Here the junction points are used within the element. For example, if the Lung has relatively less energy than the Large Intestine, IX 7 (Lu 7) is tonified to draw energy from the Large Intestine to balance the energy between the two officials. Such an imbalance can be detected on the pulses, and is known as a split pulse. Again, it is rare to find such an imbalance.

SEASONAL AND DAILY TREATMENT CYCLES

A fundamental treatment principle takes account of two natural cycles, the seasonal cycle of the year, and the daily cycle of the 24-hour clock. These treatments are carried out using points on each official, known as element points, which relate to that official's element (see Chapter 6). Here the element point combines to become both a seasonal point and a horary point. These are some of the most powerful treatments you can give, because they align the patient with the rhythms of the season and of the day.

Because the horary times for Earth, Fire and Water are during normal working hours, this is a very common treatment for patients of these elements. The horary points for Wood and Metal are during the night hours, so that it is usually only practicable to do seasonal treatments for Wood and Metal patients.

Daily treatment cycle or the Law of Midday/Midnight

This law states that in each 24-hour period each official has a period of two hours when it is at its maximum energy. This period is known as the horary time of the official. The order in which each official has its horary time is that relating to the Wei level of energy in the body, and follows the Roman

CHAPTER 9: TREATMENT PROTOCOLS

numerical order of the officials, from I to XII and back to I again. This law is also referred to as the Chinese Clock.

The law of Midday-Midnight reflects the hour by the sun, and has to be adjusted to reflect any seasonal changes when clocks may be put forward or back.

Each official also has a low period at the corresponding hours at the opposite time of the day, that is, 12 hours after the horary time. Treatment of an official during its horary time is more effective than at any other time of the day. Treatment of the horary point also has the effect of clearing out debris from an official, so that the true state of its energy can be revealed.

The horary time for each official is given in the table below:

Numeral	Official	Horary time
I	Heart	11:00 – 13:00
II	Small Intestine	13:00 – 15:00
III	Bladder	15:00 – 17:00
IV	Kidney	17:00 – 19:00
V	Heart Protector	19:00 – 21:00
VI	Three Heater	21:00 – 23:00
VII	Gall Bladder	23:00 – 01:00
VIII	Liver	01:00 – 03:00
IX	Lung	03:00 – 05:00
X	Large Intestine	05:00 – 07:00
XI	Stomach	07:00 – 09:00
XII	Spleen	09:00 – 11:00

The Law of Midday/Midnight can also be used to advise patients about how to organize their life to help the body's natural functions which are governed by the officials. If they can open their bowels during the Large Intestine's horary time of 05:00 to 07:00, food entering the stomach between 07:00 and 09:00, during the Stomach official's time, will be digested better than food eaten at any other time. Food will be digested least easily at this official's low time, between 19:00 and 21:00. Since this is when most people eat their heaviest meal, it is not surprising that people suffer from so many digestive problems.

It has also been found that giving young children chemotherapy during the Wood element's horary times, between 23:00 and 03:00 at night, helps their liver tolerate the drugs better than at any other time.

Example of a combined seasonal and horary treatment

A horary treatment on an Earth patient must be carried out between the hours of 07:00 and 11:00 to cover the period for both the Spleen and the Stomach officials. The patient is asked to come at 08:30 so that the horary point for the Stomach can be needled before 09:00 and that of the Spleen after 09:00. If this treatment is carried out during Late Summer, Earth's season, it will become one of the most powerful treatments to give an Earth patient.

CHAPTER 10

POINT SELECTION

Guidelines for selecting points
List of my favourite points for each element
Example of point selection for first four treatments

GUIDELINES FOR SELECTING POINTS

We must always remember that points are servants of the elements, never their masters. The power they have is handed to them by the elements whose instructions they obey and whose energy they serve. Isolated from the elements, they are powerless. Therefore in looking at this list of points, always keep in mind the power of the elements in whose service they work.

We must also try not to allow ourselves to become confused by the thought of the 365 possible points from which to select our treatment, but break this selection down into the smaller groupings some of which I have already discussed in previous chapters.

By far the most important groups of points for a five element acupuncturist are the following:

- Command points
- Points used to clear blocks

Armed with these points alone, a newly qualified practitioner with no experience to draw upon will be able to treat his/her patients very successfully and, most importantly, very safely.

We now need to look at one of the most complex areas of point selection. What points in addition to the ones in the groups I have already mentioned do we need to add to enhance the effects of our treatments? To help us make what is always a difficult choice, the selection of one from many other possible points, we can draw not only upon what those with more experience have told us, or on what we have learnt from our own experience, but also on the names of points and their anatomical location, as helpful pointers for our choices. Both name and location will add to our understanding of the significance of a point. If we look at the meridian system as a map in this way, we can regard each point as providing a signpost by which to orientate ourselves and help us take our bearings.

In five element acupuncture, more than in many other branches of acupuncture, the emphasis we place upon treating an element through its officials makes the task of more complex point selection surprisingly easy, provided that we do not allow ourselves to become confused by the many books listing acupuncture points for their individual function, rather than their function as servants of the elements. To make a five element acupuncturist's life as simple as possible where point selection is concerned, we need always remember that the aim of choosing any point is to enhance an element's balance. The simplest way to do this is to choose points on the meridians of its two officials, or points on other meridians which relate specifically to its officials, such as AEPs or alarm points. There are, however, some points whose effect is not limited to one element, but which add energy and balance to all the elements (those listed in Groups 2 and 3 below).

Here to help us, it is useful to think of points as belonging to four different groups:

Group 1: Points on an element's officials to be used <u>at any stage of treatment</u>

a. Command points (see Chapter 6)

b. A small group of three points which can be added to command point level points very early on in treatment to stir the respective official into action. These points are:

For the Earth element:

- **XII 8 (Sp 8) Earth Motivator:** I see XII 8 as being a kind of excavator helping to churn over the earth when it has become heavy and clay-like. It should be thought of at the start of their treatment for Earth people who seem to be very stuck as a way of helping the element to move.

- **XI 24 (St 24) Lubrication Food Gate:** This is like a sister point to XII 8, and can be considered early on in treatment if you feel that your patient's Earth element has the consistency of shifting sand rather than heavy clay, which would point to XII 8 instead. It gives the necessary lubrication to Earth to enable food to be processed properly.

CHAPTER 10: POINT SELECTION

For the Metal element:

- **IX 8 (Lu 8) Meridian Gutter:** We will consider adding this point very early on to help the Metal element clear away the rubbish to allow the Lung to breathe in fresh air.

c. Points to be used to clear blocks (see Chapter 7)

Group 2: Points not on an element's officials which can be used for all elements early on in treatment

Apart from Group 1 points, these are additional points which can be added to the first few treatments when you feel that a patient's energy needs the extra boost each of these points can give. It is important that you do not routinely add one of these points, but consider carefully the patient's needs, and only add a point if this seems necessary. Experience will gradually help you in deciding whether you need to add one of these points, and which one to choose. Here, the point names can also themselves be used as indicators of what each point can offer a patient.

CV 8 Spirit Deficiency and CV 14 Great Deficiency

CV 8 is a point which can be used in the first few treatments as well as at any stage of treatment if you feel that the patient is low in spirit. It is never needled because of its position at the centre of the umbilicus, but used only with moxibustion (on a base of salt) (see Chapter 8 for details of the procedure to be used).

CV 14 can be used instead if the patient's blood pressure is too high to allow moxibustion. Because CV 14 is the alarm point of the Heart, I like to think that it has a slightly greater effect on the spirit than CV 8. It can also be used later on in treatment as a follow-up to treatment with CV 8.

IV 24 (Ki 24) Spirit Burial Ground

As its name indicates, this is very much a point to consider when you feel that a person's spirit is buried or dead to them. This point will help resuscitate the spirit deep within. The need for it will often appear in eyes which seem lifeless. The Kidney provides our reserves of energy, and we can only draw on the reserves from the other five Kidney chest points when they have been built up sufficiently during the first stages of treatment to provide something to offer other elements. The other Kidney chest points are therefore only used later on in treatment.

III 37 (Bl 42) Soul Door
This point lies at the same horizontal level as the AEP of the Lung, and therefore has a close association with the Metal element, and the Lung in particular. As the name of the point indicates, this opens up a door to the spirit.

III 38 (Bl 43) Rich for the Vitals
This point lies at the same horizontal level as the AEP of the Heart Protector, and therefore has a close association with the Fire element and Outer Fire in particular. Because of the Heart Protector's control over blood circulation, it is used to help nourish the blood, and can be used early on in treatment if the patient seems very anaemic. J.R. Worsley said that, like blood, this point reaches every cell in the body, and it therefore has many uses at different stages of treatment.

It is one of the few points in five element acupuncture which can be needled repeatedly. It is excellent for helping patients who are undergoing chemo- or radiotherapy, where the number of moxas can be increased by increments of 7 from treatment to treatment (7 to start with, followed by 14, 21 up to a total of 50 moxas on each side).

III 39 (Bl 44) Spirit Hall
This point lies at the same horizontal level as the AEP of the Heart, and therefore also has a close association with the Fire Element and with Inner Fire in particular. As the name of the point indicates, this allows the patient's spirit to wander through the hall of the spirit. It can be used later on in treatment after the door to the spirit, III 37 (Bl 42), has been needled.

It is a difficult clinical judgement to decide whether a patient needs III 37 Soul Door or III 39 Spirit Hall to nourish their spirit. The association with either Metal or Fire can help decide which point would be more appropriate.

Group 3: Points not on an element's officials which can be used for all elements <u>at later stages of treatment</u>
These include all CV and GV, Outer Bladder and Kidney chest points, plus one other point, Heart 1.

I 1 (Ht 1) Utmost Source
Here, this point's name helps define its function, for it connects the Heart to the source of all things, to the great worlds beyond us, to Heaven in its widest sense. It can be used to help those who feel cut off from communication at

a deep level with their fellow human beings, as though they live in isolation from the world in which they live. It is one of the points which is not just restricted to supporting Inner Fire, but can be used to help all the officials.

If we think of its position on the body, this point is at the apex of the meridian's pathway, and is the entry point to the superficial pathway of the Heart official. Interestingly enough, to needle this point, we have to ask the patient to raise the arm to expose the armpit and open up the point to the needle, almost as though we are asking the patient to raise their arms to the Heaven above. It is to this point that the energies of Heaven pour down to us from above, acting as a true connecting point to what lies above and beyond us. Needling this point ensures that the connection to Heaven remains open and available to a patient.

Group 4: Non-command points on an element's officials to be used later on in treatment

I give below my own selection of these points. They are ones which I feel confident to use and use regularly. When I choose any of these, I feel that I am like some craftsman of the spirit, turning to a few well-tried, well-beloved tools of my trade. This list should not be seen as prescriptive, and is meant to help the novice practitioner over one of the great hurdles they experience, which is their worry about points.

Each practitioner will build up their own repertoire of points as their experience increases. I use a surprisingly small repertoire of under 60 points in addition to the ones in the different groups listed above. Other practitioners may use many different ones, and perhaps more of them. The important thing here is that each practitioner should feel confident in their selection, since this confidence and trust in the points they select will feed its way through to the treatment, and make it more effective.

I make no apology for quoting here some of the many comments about individual points which I heard J.R. Worsley make. I am still astonished by his profound insights into the individual qualities of the points he talked about. I was fortunate to hear him going through the full list of 365 points point by point, addressing each of them as though they were close friends with whom he communicated at a level I can only aspire to from a distance.

Some of the points in this group will also be used as command points or to clear blocks. They are included here when I select them for the spirit of what they offer. Implicit within any point is its relationship to the name it bears, and every point, including command points, can therefore be selected for its spirit as well as for its function. Thus V 8 (HP 8), Palace of Weariness, which is the Fire point of a Fire official, and becomes a horary or seasonal point at the correct time, can be selected for its ability to provide a warm haven in which the patient's weary spirit can shelter. It can do this at any time and in any season, and it will always bring with it some of the warmth that a Fire point within a Fire official has within it, although not as intensely as at Fire time in summer.

It is worth remembering that yang officials all have many more points to choose from than their yin companions, and this is reflected in my list. My choice of point is influenced by my own perception of the difference between yin and yang officials. I see the yin as being reservoirs for the particular quality of an element's energy, controlling the release of this energy as though from within some command control, whilst the yang act as their messengers, distributing their commands round the body. A yin official can therefore be regarded as a queen bee at the centre of an element's hive, and the yang as the worker bees sent out to deliver the queen's instructions. When choosing possible points on an element, you may therefore like to consider whether it is more important to give your patient more of the quality of its yin or its yang official. Of course, this is a difficult choice to make, but nothing relating to point selection is easy.

It is also important to remove some of the burden of trying to make the 'right' point selection, as there is no such thing. Who is really to say whether an Earth patient today who appears distressed will benefit from the point XI 19 (St 19), which we call Not at Ease, rather than from XI 25 (St 25), Heavenly Pivot? How are we to decide whether it is more important that we first reduce some of their unease with XI 19 or centre them more firmly with XI 25, since this will also reduce their unease but by a different route? I suggest that both are as effective as each other, becoming so when the practitioner selecting one or other is sure that this point satisfies more closely his/her patient's needs than the other point. Another practitioner might choose quite a different point altogether, such as XI 40 (St 40) Abundant Splendour, thinking, equally correctly, that any Earth person's distress will be helped by being given the radiant warmth this point can bestow.

Finally, a note of warning here. I think it makes for sloppy practice if you rely for your point selection too much on the names of points. This tends to make you dart around all over the meridians searching for points whose names you like, perhaps forgetting whilst you are doing this that good five element treatment does not come from the choice of points but from the right choice of element.

LIST OF MY FAVOURITE POINTS FOR EACH ELEMENT

The Windows of the Sky must also be included in this group of points (see Chapter 6).

Wood points
Liver (VIII)

VIII 13 Chapter Gate and VIII 14 Gate of Hope

It is interesting that the Liver has two gates, one next to the other, almost as though it may need these two openings together to help the Wood element burst through. There is a lovely tape I once heard of J.R. Worsley talking about how the Gate of Hope stretches out its branches, just as a tree does, to reach up to find the air above its head given it by the first point of the Lung lying directly above. When I clear a VIII/IX block, I always have this image of my treatment helping the spreading branches of a tree to draw in the sustenance from the heavens above without which it will wither and die.

These two points can be needled together, first VIII 13 and then VIII 14 for maximum effect, but I have tended to concentrate just on opening the Gate of Hope. We can think of VIII 13 as helping to open a new chapter in a patient's life, and of VIII 14 as providing the hope without which the Liver can make no future plans.

Gall Bladder (VII)

VII 20 Wind Pond

Here I have the corroboration of something one of my Wood patients told me which I have never forgotten. She loved having this point needled because she could immediately feel the tight muscles of her upper neck relaxing, allowing her to move her head freely. All points around the neck are extremely important because this is where an official's energy is gathered closely together after travelling up over the trunk of the body before bursting up into the head. It is not surprising, therefore, that there are so many Windows of the Sky in this most important area of the body.

VII 24 Sun and Moon

We were told that we should wait a little in our Wood treatments, and use this point a little later on to harmonize the Wood element, just as bringing sun and moon together is like recreating the harmony of the Dao.

VII 25 Capital Gate

Another gate for the Wood element, lying anatomically close to VIII 13 Chapter Gate.

Fire points: Inner Fire
Heart (I)

I 1 Utmost Source

See Group 3 points above.

I 5 Penetrating Inside

This is the junction point which joins the Heart to its companion official, the Small Intestine. I see it as helping bring the energy from the Heart deep inside to feed the Small Intestine, and drawing energy from the Small Intestine back down into the Heart. I therefore sometimes finish treatment on the Small Intestine by adding this point on the Heart official.

These are the only two points of the Heart official that I use, apart from command points. The Japanese, we were told, never needle the Heart Meridian because they view it as a sacred official. Since the Japanese all learnt originally from Chinese masters, this forms part of a longstanding Chinese tradition which emphasizes great respect for the Heart.

Small Intestine (II)

II 9–II 15

Of the Small Intestine's 19 points, perhaps the most important group, apart from the command points, are those on the back, points II 9–II 15, which criss-cross the scapula. Whilst GV and Inner and Outer Bladder points follow the line of the spine, and thus act as support for the almost immobile vertical axis of the body, the Small Intestine controls the two wings of the scapula which provide mobility for the back and for the head as it pivots on the neck. The scapula is the only part of the back which can move independently of the spine.

II 9 can be regarded as the yang equivalent of I 1. It lies on the same plane but on the yang, posterior aspect of the armpit, as opposed to its yin, anterior aspect. It is a good point to use to strengthen the Small Intestine as it starts its climb up and over the scapula. The other points on the back can be used at different times to add to the work of II 9, with II 14 and II 15, which lie closest to the spine, giving an extra level of vertical support to the GV line.

CHAPTER 10: POINT SELECTION

Fire points: Outer Fire
Heart Protector (V)

V 4 Gate of Qi Reserve

This point is often paired with VI 7 Assembly of Ancestors. I like to think that V 4 opens a gate into the reserves of the Heart which it is the Heart Protector's function to protect, and VI 7 adds to those reserves all the power which the ancestors pass on to their descendants. That is why I like needling V 4 first, followed by VI 7, rather than the usual order of yang before yin.

V 8 Palace of Weariness

Here we are not thinking of it as a horary/seasonal point, but to help those who are weary in spirit find comfort and strength.

Three Heater (VI)

VI 10 Heavenly Well

I remember J.R. Worsley saying that this is a 'much under-used point', so I use it a lot because of that! It is, of course, the Earth point on the Three Heater, and therefore provides the kind of foundation which Earth always gives to every official. Each point with a name associated with heaven has that something extra which comes to our spirit from above. As I needle it, I like to think of my needle as a bucket going deep down into this spiritual well. It gives me something of the same feeling as needling V 4 Gate of Qi Reserve.

VI 18 Feeding Meridians

One of the Three Heater's functions is to harmonize everything and make what is needed available to all the officials. It therefore supports the actions of every other official. Basing my thinking on the name of this point, I use it to help the Three Heater in this task.

VI 23 Silk Bamboo Hollow

We needle VI 22, the point immediately before it on the meridian, because it is the meridian's exit point and therefore often used to clear an Entry-Exit block. That leaves this one point beyond it, VI 23, almost as though it is not part of the Three Heater meridian, and yet it should by rights be the exit point, since it lies immediately above the entry point of the Gall Bladder, VII 1, on the lateral canthus of the eye. As with all things to do with the location of points, this is another one of those oddities which make acupuncture so fascinating.

Its position as the final point of the Three Heater meridian, added to its name, which makes us think of the hollow space inside a bamboo stalk, makes me see this point as being an opening from outside to inside, bringing welcome warmth and harmony deep within to body and soul.

Earth points
Spleen (XII)

XII 4 Prince's Grandson

We were always encouraged to use this point in combination with XI 40 Abundant Splendour (see below). A Prince's Grandson was considered to be so important because he was there to carry on the royal lineage.

XII 15 Great Horizontal

This point is used in combination with XI 25 Heavenly Pivot. Both lie on the same horizontal line as CV 8, and form part of the line of points including IV 16 which can be regarded as allowing us to pivot around our centre. These two points therefore ensure that Earth feels properly centred.

XII 20 Encircling Glory

I love this point, not only for its name, but for where it lies. I feel when I am needling it that I am enfolding my Earth patients within a circle of warmth.

XII 21 Great Enveloping

This point is often used to clear an Entry-Exit block, but can also be used much as I use XII 20 above. Both points encourage the feeling that you are enclosing Earth in a warm embrace.

Stomach (XI)

XI 4 Earth Granary

This point provides a granary where Earth can store the food it takes in. Its position at the corner of the mouth is a good pointer to how it can be used. When I have needled this point, Earth patients who often continue talking whilst I am treating them (inability to stop processing) have suddenly fallen silent in mid-sentence as their Stomach is at last able to swallow their thoughts.

XI 8 Head Tied

As its name indicates, this is a very useful point indeed for helping an Earth patient whose head is constantly churning over with thoughts. It is not easy to locate, but I find it by drawing a straight line up from the outer canthus of the eye stopping just slightly in from the hairline.

XI 12 Broken Bowl

If a bowl is cracked, everything drains out. In the same way, an Earth person can feel as though things constantly drain from them, however much they take in. This point helps seal the cracks to ensure that the food they take in by both body and soul is available to nourish themselves and others.

XI 19 Not at Ease

Earth can often seem uneasy and dissatisfied, and this is a point to consider here. It is on the same horizontal plane as CV 14 Great Deficiency, the alarm point of the Heart, and I like to think that, because of this, it takes on some of CV 14's power.

XI 24 Lubrication Food Gate

See Group 1b above.

XI 25 Heavenly Pivot

See note on XII 15 above.

XI 37 Upper Great Void and XI 39 Lower Great Void

It is good to think of these points as a pair, although they can be used individually. Earth can feel very empty, as though starving, and one or other or both of these points can be considered for patients who seem undernourished in spirit. You have to make a judgement as to which area of the body is creating this feeling of emptiness. Is it the upper part, which relates more to the spirit, an inability to feed the spirit, in which case you choose XI 37, or the lower part, which relates more to physical emptiness, an inability to feed the body, in which case you will choose XI 39? If the patient feels totally depleted, then both points can be needled together at the same treatment.

XI 40 Abundant Splendour

XI 40's name is self-explanatory. Which Earth person would not like an abundant harvest? See also its associated point, XII 4 above.

Metal points
Lung (IX)

IX 1 Middle Palace

This is the point towards which VIII 14 Gate of Hope stretches out, the first point of the Lung, a central Palace and a place fit for an Emperor. I remember J.R. Worsley recommending for a Metal patient of mine that I should do IX 1 first, followed by IX 2 at the next treatment, and finally IX 3, the Lung's Window of the Sky, at the treatment after that. This was the first time that I became aware of the fact that we can think of the points as being in a progression starting from the first point and moving up or down the meridian, and that this progression can form part of treatment.

IX 2 Cloud Gate

IX 2 is the next point in this climb up the Lung official, a gate which opens the clouds above our heads to let light and air through. We were told that we can also use this point to draw clouds down to obscure a sun which shines too brightly. It was fascinating to hear that points could have this dual role. Do not ask your patient to breathe in when you needle IX 1 or IX 2, as both lie directly over the lung and you have to be careful to needle only to the depth allowed.

IX 8 Meridian Gutter

See Group 1b above.

IX 10 Fish Region

J.R. Worsley called this 'the most spiritual point in the body'. I use this as a way not only of bringing this quality to Metal patients, but of seeing whether I am on the right element. I always tell a patient what J.R. told me, and then I watch for the patient's reactions. All Metal patients, without fail, understand immediately what I mean and show by their reaction that they feel that they are privileged to receive what this point has to offer. Patients of other elements react quite differently, some with incomprehension, some with puzzlement, some with no interest whatsoever. So if you are in doubt about whether your patient is Metal, do as I do, and use this point to help in your diagnosis. We need all the help we can.

This is one of the rare cases where I talk to patients about the points I am using. Usually I don't, on the understanding that a patient isn't there to study acupuncture, but to get better.

Large Intestine (X)

X 7 Warm Current

I like to think of this point as bringing warmth to what can often be a rather chilly element.

I am aware of how few additional Large Intestine points I use. I appear instead to concentrate much more on helping the Lung, on the principle that it is essential to focus on helping it in its task of taking in and providing inspiration, in the deepest sense of the word, for body and soul.

Water points
Kidney (IV)

IV 1 Bubbling Spring

I think this is a much under-used point, probably because of its position right in the centre of the sole of the foot, and, very much like V 8, a very painful point to needle. This may be why practitioners seem either to avoid it or not think of it at all. Its under-use may also be because it is better to needle it with the patient lying on their stomach to expose the sole of the foot, and I have found that people often avoid points where they have to turn patients over or round in this way, a tendency to laziness in practitioners which we should all be aware of. I have had confirmation that it is well named from patients who have told me that it feels 'like a fountain of water rushing up my leg'.

Like Heart 1, the first point on a meridian holds a special place in that meridian's functions. Here I see this point as connecting the Water element to the ground beneath our feet, and thus able to draw up the Earth's energy into the body.

IV 2 Blazing Valley

J.R. Worsley said that it was good to follow IV 1 with the Fire point of the Kidney, thereby warming up the flow of Water on its way up the body. I always couple IV 2 with III 60 (Bl 60) Kunlun Mountains, the Fire point of the Bladder, since I think it must be good for both Water officials to receive Fire's warmth in this way.

IV 16 Vitals Correspondence

I was told that this point was like the III 38 (Bl 43) of the Kidney. I interpreted this as meaning a point which has a very wide function, with a very widespread range of uses, as III 38 has. Because of its position at the same horizontal level as CV 8 and XI 25 (St 25), I also see this as a balancing point for the Kidney, being on the central axis of the body and thus contributing to maintaining balance.

IV 24 Spirit Burial Ground
See Group 2 points above.

IV 25 Spirit Storehouse and IV 27 Store House
Obviously a storehouse of the spirit is a deeper point than a simple store house, which is shown by their anatomical location. IV 25 lies very close to the Heart, whilst IV 27 is closer to the clavicle. You should only consider these points once you are sure that treatment has built up sufficient energy in the Kidney to be drawn upon by needling these points. Ask yourself whether you think there is enough in the store to feed the other officials. Neither point should therefore be used early on in treatment.

Bladder (III): Inner Bladder Line

III 60 Kunlun Mountains (with IV 2, as mentioned above)
As with IV 2, this warms up the flow of Water on its way up the body.

Bladder (III): Outer Bladder Line

III 37–39 (42–44)
See Group 2 points above.

III 44 Thought Dwelling and III 45 Stomach Granary
Both are at the level of the AEPs of the Earth element, and, as their names suggest, both have a strong connection to the Earth element. If you want to add something of the depth of an Outer Bladder point to an Earth patient, then one of these is a point I would consider. You might make your choice by deciding whether this patient needs help with processing thoughts or with digesting food.

III 42 Spiritual Soul Gate
I always treat this point with respect ever since I heard J.R. Worsley saying that it is 'deeper than IV 24'. If the spirit is not resuscitated by Spirit Burial Ground, then we should go to the deeper level of the spirit at Spiritual Soul Gate.

III 47 Ambition Room

When I think it is important for a patient to have deeper aspirations for their life, I select this point, telling them what J.R. Worsley told us, 'Everybody has to have an ambition. It doesn't matter at all if you change it the next day, but you have to have one for today.' Patients seem to understand and love this. This is another of the few occasions when I tell patients something about a point, as with IX 10 (Lu 10).

Conception Vessel (CV) and Governor Vessel (GV)

Unlike any other group of points relating to a particular meridian, all CV and GV points can be used for any official. The difficulty then is how to select which point will be useful from the total of 52 points (24 CV and 28 GV). Some of these points are forbidden to use at all, others forbidden either to needle or to add moxa, so you need to look up in a point reference chart to see which these are.

Even though Governor Vessel moves upward from GV 1 over the top of the head, for some reason I like to think of the GV points in reverse order, starting at the top and moving down over the back, whereas I do the opposite with CV points. This is an oddity I have never quite worked out the reason for, but may well be that I like to think of GV as receiving its strength from Heaven, and CV its strength from the Earth below our feet.

I am giving you below a few tips to help you choose from amongst this bewildering profusion of points:

1. You need to distinguish between what a yin official offers (CV) and what a yang official offers (GV). Yang officials provide the outer defences of an official, yin look after its inner core. GV is therefore the official of choice literally and figuratively for strengthening a patient's backbone, for holding the body and soul's outer structure in place to allow CV to come to the aid of our inner structure deep within. Which of these two aspects do you think your patient needs today?

2. You can call upon your understanding of the three jiao to help you. Remember which officials lie within the areas covered by the upper, the middle or the lower jiao. If you are trying to help the Fire or Metal elements, it is more appropriate to think of CV/GV points on the areas of back and front under the control of the upper jiao. With Wood and Earth we will think of the middle jiao, which relates to organs of processing. The lower jiao has a close relationship to the Water element, Fire (II) and Metal (X).

3. Remember the alarm points for each official, and where they are. The majority are CV points, and will therefore guide you to use these points for their associated official. The exceptions are the two alarm points for the Wood and Metal elements, but their anatomical locations will be another pointer as to where along the CV or GV line you may make your choice.

4. You can also think of the anatomical position of the AEPs of a patient's element, and relate your choice of CV or GV point to the horizontal line corresponding to these AEPs (for instance, GV 12 to the AEP of the Lung, or GV 8 to the AEP of the Liver). This is easier when choosing GV points which are on the back, but you can also think of the corresponding horizontal position for the CV points on the front as a kind of rough guide.

Conception Vessel

CV 8 Spirit Deficiency and CV 14 Great Deficiency
See Group 2 above.

CV 22 Heaven Rushing Out
This point is CV's Window of the Sky, and I like to use this particularly when the patient has problems around the neck area, such as problems in swallowing, or for those with thyroid imbalances, and I feel that they need the additional strength CV gives to element treatment. It can be found by placing one finger below the cricoid cartilage and another at the top. The point is ⅓ of the way up.

Governor Vessel

GV 20 One Hundred Meetings
This point and GV 21 lie at the topmost point of the body, and I choose GV 20 rather than GV 21 because it is also a Dragon point, and I like to think that it therefore has a depth to it which GV 21 does not. I have used GV 20 as a point for anybody who has odd feelings of discomfort in the head, or had surgery on the head. Patients have told me that they feel a lovely shower of sparkling energy pouring over their head right down their body. Emotionally, too, it will help somebody whose head is as though whirring with thoughts and emotions, and I find it then has a very calming effect. To locate it, practise on yourself until you come to a slight soft dip in the skin. When you palpate this gently you begin to feel a strong tingling which will become unpleasant

if you do it for too long. It's not an easy point to find, but I have learnt to locate it by this method.

GV 14 Great Hammer

This point can be needled first followed by the AEPs when a patient is not improving and is as though stuck. The Great Hammer will give the two officials a jolt to enable the AEPs to do their work.

GV 13 Kiln Path

Kilns are a kind of oven, so I see this point as warming the GV meridian.

GV 12 Body Pillar

A rather over-used point, in my opinion. It is as though practitioners are glad to have a point with a name they can relate to, and one which it is also easy to locate, being at the level of the Lung AEPs. You don't want to use it early on in treatment, as I have seen done too many times, because you want to assess whether the officials have enough strength in themselves to hold the body (and soul) upright. Only use this point if you feel that body and soul are crumbling despite work on the patient's element.

GV 8 Contracted Muscle

This point lies on the same horizontal axis as the AEP of the Liver, and the Wood element is all to do with control of muscular movement. This is therefore an excellent point for Wood patients whose tendons and ligaments are tight and 'contracted', but can be used, of course, where there is a taut back for any element, as all CV and GV points can be used for any element.

EXAMPLE OF POINT SELECTION FOR FIRST FOUR TREATMENTS

Treatment 1

1. Check for possession/clear if present
2. AE drain
3. Source points of the guardian element

NB: If possible the centre pulse and the Akabanes should have been corrected at the time of the Physical Diagnosis at the end of the TD. If this has not been possible, these should be done at the end of Treatment 1, unless the Possession and AE drain takes too long. In that case, it should be done at the start of Treatment 2.

Treatment 2

At the start of each treatment from now on check for H/W and/or E/E blocks as a routine procedure, before moving on to other treatment.

1. One point from Group 2 points, but only if considered necessary
2. Tonification points

Treatment 3

1. Again add one point from Group 2, but only if considered necessary, or if you think the patient's element is either Earth or Metal, you might feel it appropriate to add one of the three points listed in Group 1b for these two elements.
2. If possible horary or seasonal treatment, and ideally horary and seasonal treatment at the right horary and seasonal time. If not, then either source or tonification points.

Treatment 4

1. AEPs
2. Source, tonification or transfer points

I have made a deliberately simple selection of points for these four treatments. Many five element acupuncturists will want to add one (or even more) points from Group 2 as an automatic addition, something I try to advise a beginner against. I want to emphasize again how important it is to learn the craft of five element acupuncture using the simplest tools to start with. By adding more complex point selection at an early stage, you may not learn to recognize the effectiveness of command points on their own, and this will be doing your patients a great disservice.

A word of advice: Do not fall into the habit of changing the element you have chosen until you have directed at least four treatments at it. If you then feel that nothing much is changing, it will be time to move on, but also giving the new element you choose four treatments. If you move away from one element to another too quickly you will never be sure whether you stayed long enough on an element to allow treatment a chance to work.

Once you feel confident that treatment is progressing as it should, you can start including some of the points listed in Groups 3 and 4.

Postscript

What has gone before touches mainly upon those outward manifestations of our practice, the skills and techniques needed to select an appropriate treatment and needle the points appropriately. It can naturally do no more than skim the surface of what five element practice is about, for to what I have written here we have to add our patients who come to us each with their unique and complex needs. Such is the depth of each human being that to presume to offer them our help is always somewhat audacious, a daring attempt to alter the course of another's life, however subtly and with however honest an intention, and we have to engage in such a potentially profound encounter with humility.

Some of us would prefer instead to dwell on those aspects of their practice which have about them always a tinge of the almost exclusively physical, reminiscent of much Western medical practice. Five element acupuncture, too, can remain on the surface in this way, if its practitioner feels uneasy at plunging the depths of the soul which lie hidden within the physical envelope of our bodies. But I feel it is doing our patients the utmost disservice, is indeed unethical in its deepest sense, if we have been given, in the elements, an understanding of the powerful forces of body and soul hidden within each of us and yet choose not to make use of this in our practice. For the elements open up to us the landscape of the soul, with all its deep inadequacies, its longings and its potential for profound inner development and fulfilment.

Who cannot be awed at being invited by each of our patients to walk through this profound landscape with them?

APPENDIX

TEACH YOURSELF MANUAL

Contents

How to use this manual — 147

Lesson 1 — 148
  Introduction to the elements
  Roman numerals
  Pulse-taking
  Reference cards

Lesson 2 — 150
  The Wood element
  Blood pressure
  Three jiao

Lesson 3 — 152
  The Fire element
  Alarm points
  Centre pulse
  Pulse-taking notation

Lesson 4 — 155
  The Earth element
  Akabane test
  Touch

Lesson 5 — 158
  The Metal element
  Physical Diagnosis
  Importance of touch

Lesson 6 — 161
  The Water element
  Physical Diagnosis

Lesson 7 — 163
  The Traditional Diagnosis (TD)
  Patient-practitioner relationship
  Level of imbalance
  Causes of disease

Lesson 8 — 165
- Sensory and emotional signatures
- Training our senses: colour
- Acupuncture points

Lesson 9 — 167
- Sound of voice
- Law of Mother-Child and Sheng and Ke cycles
- Tonification, sedation and energy transfers

Lesson 10 — 169
- Training our senses: smell
- Aggressive Energy (AE)
- Associated Effect Points (AEPs)
- Needling techniques

Lesson 11 — 171
- Training our senses: emotion
- Point selection
- Seasonal and daily treatment cycles
- Treatment techniques: moxibustion

Lesson 12 — 173
- The different stages of treatment
- Selection of element

Lesson 13 — 175
- Possession
- Assessing the effects of treatment
- Law of Cure

Lesson 14 — 177
- The Law of Husband-Wife
- Entry-Exit blocks
- Blocks caused by scars
- Example of point selection for first four treatments

Lesson 15 — 179
- Windows of the Sky
- Further guidelines for selecting points

Lesson 16 — 180
- Spacing of treatments
- Patient's role in treatment

Conclusion — 181

How to Use This Manual

The following lessons refer to chapters and sections in the Handbook.

Although this self-help manual is suitable for people who need to work on their own, a group of people working together will find that their learning will be helped if they are able to work through the lessons with others. This will only be possible where there are enough acupuncturists or those interested in acupuncture to gather together. As I know, many people live in geographically isolated areas, with no access to fellow acupuncturists, or no acupuncturists near them at all. It is these people, in particular, who have spurred me on to write these lessons.

Most of the lessons are divided into two sections. The first lists the relevant chapters and sections in the Handbook to be read, and the second covers practical work to help develop specific skills. Only trained acupuncturists will be able to do some of the practical exercises I have suggested for each lesson, such as those relating to needling or point location, but there are other practical exercises which the lay person can be interested to try their hand at.

MY BLOGS

It will also be helpful for you to read posts from my two blogs on topics which relate to what you are studying. The blogs complement what is in the lessons and will add to your understanding. Of particular interest for those just starting to treat will be the posts in my Five Element Treatment blog, which cover actual treatments I have given my patients. These will help you begin to understand the reasoning behind the choice of points for specific treatments.

www.norafranglen.blogspot.com

www.five-element-treatments.blogspot.co.uk

LESSON 1

Introduction to the elements
Roman numerals
Pulse-taking
Reference cards

A. READING FROM THE HANDBOOK

1. Read the Handbook slowly from cover to cover. This will give you an overview of what you will be learning. Don't try to learn anything – just get a feeling for the different topics. You will be looking in detail at each topic in the different lessons.

2. Then go back and re-read the Introduction and Chapter 1, 'The Five Elements'. These form a general introduction to an approach to the elements.

3. Re-read the Postscript at the end of the Handbook. What I have written there is the most important statement in the Handbook. Everything we do as five element acupuncturists must be directed at helping heal a patient's spirit, not just their body.

B. PRACTICAL WORK

1. Read the 'Five elements and their 12 officials' section in Chapter 2. Learn the Roman numerals for the officials.

2. Read the 'Pulse-taking' section in Chapter 4. Practise taking pulses in the five element way. The best way for you to take them is on somebody lying down. If this is not possible, you will have to take pulses with the person sitting on a chair. Remember that it is important to hold the patient's hand with both of your hands as shown, and to hold their hand against your body so that you are making close contact.

   Start by taking the pulses of five people a day, and then increase this gradually. Don't worry about trying to interpret what you are feeling, and don't try and write anything down. Just let your fingers get used to taking the pulses, and let the elements start talking to you through your touch on the patient's pulses. You will move on to writing pulse pictures down when you are a little more familiar with taking pulses.

Remember that you are approaching a person at a very deep level when you palpate their pulses, so be gentle with your touch. People should give you feedback if they feel you are pressing too heavily.

3. Reference cards: Buy a plastic photo album with plastic sleeves as a card index to use as reference in the practice room. Complete a card for the Roman numerals and for the different pulse positions. It does not look professional if you need to refer to the Handbook when treating patients, but it is easy to look quickly at the reference cards. Prepare to write individual cards to help memorize points and procedures for different topics as you go through this course of lessons.

Lesson 2

The Wood element
Blood pressure
Three jiao

A. READING FROM THE HANDBOOK

1. Read the 'Introduction to the elements' section in Chapter 2.
2. Read the 'Wood element' section in Chapter 2.
3. Learn the list of Wood's characteristics, including:
   - Wood's organs: the Gall Bladder (yang) and the Liver (yin)
   - Wood's colour, sound, smell and emotion
   - Wood's season and time of day

Then think about Wood in nature. If you are lucky enough to do this in Wood's season, spring, all you need do is to walk outside and let what is going on outside flow into you. If you are trying to experience Wood in another season, then picture a time when you have walked outside in nature in spring. Ask yourself what is happening around you and how this makes you feel. Because spring is a slow season to develop, you have plenty of time to feel spring's changing energy as it goes from the first stirrings of buds in the earth to the moment when the buds burst forth into flower or leaf.

Try to relate what you observe in nature to human activity. One of the easiest ways of doing this is to look at some famous people on the internet or television. Short video extracts are an ideal way of doing this, because they are often selected for very characteristic or extreme behaviour. The list below gives some Wood people to look out for:

Margaret Thatcher, George Bush, Boris Becker, Wayne Rooney, Queen Elizabeth, Princess Anne, Queen Victoria, Rafael Nadal

Look at each clip several times, and try and match what you see to some of the energy in nature in springtime. Observe how energetic all the people seem to be, with strong voices and quick movements. Try to observe what these people have in common which makes us think these may be Wood people.

Then start applying anything you have learnt so far about the Wood element to people you know personally, such as your family, friends or colleagues. You may be surprised how quickly you begin to see that a particular person has a characteristic of speech, behaviour or body movement which reminds you of one of the famous people you have been looking at. If so, watch them carefully as they go about their normal life, and then look again at a video clip of the famous person they may remind you of, trying to see what both have in common.

Whilst you are doing all this, do not forget the signs of the Wood element in yourself. What do you feel like when you get angry, for example? Think of a situation when somebody or something made you very angry. Try and feel this anger in your body, and you will see that it begins to stiffen, as if the muscles are tightening. You will find your mouth clamping shut, and your hands turning into fists, as if you are getting ready to fight. You will probably feel as if everything inside you is active and about to spring forward. Then imagine what it must be like to be a Wood person (you may be one yourself!) in whom every action is like this. If you can begin to feel how this energy does its work inside you, then you are on the way to understanding a little more what it is like to be of the Wood element.

Don't move away from the Wood element to the Fire element until you feel you have got some idea of some of its qualities through doing as I suggest above. It is better not to be overwhelmed by information about more than one element at a time at this stage of your learning. There is no hurry at all in this. The longer you take to absorb some of the characteristics of an element, the more you will begin to see it in the people around you, and of course in yourself, too. Once you feel you are ready, but only then, you may feel you want to move on to the Fire element, the child of Wood.

B. PRACTICAL WORK

1. Read the 'Blood pressure' section in Chapter 4. Take the blood pressure of a few people, and write down whether the blood pressure is in the normal or abnormal range, and therefore whether moxibustion should or should not be added before needling.

2. Read the 'Three jiao' section in Chapter 4. Practise feeling the temperature of the three jiao on some people, and write down what you feel in the way described.

Lesson 3

The Fire element
Alarm points
Centre pulse
Pulse-taking notation

A. READING FROM THE HANDBOOK

1. Read the 'Fire element' section in Chapter 2, with its two aspects, Inner and Outer Fire.

2. Learn the list of Fire's characteristics, including:

   - Fire's organs and functions:
     - Inner Fire: the Small Intestine (yang) and the Heart (yin)
     - Outer Fire: the Three Heater (yang) and the Heart Protector (yin)
   - Fire's colour, sound, smell and emotion
   - Fire's season and times of day

Think about the summer time. Even if you are doing this in another season, remember how you feel in the heat of summer, and relate this to what can go on inside a Fire person. Their Fire may be just at a pleasant level and warm you when you come into contact with it, or over-heat and become so hot that it burns you when you go near it. When you are treating a Fire person, you are trying to make sure that the natural warmth of the Heart within them remains balanced, neither too hot nor too cold, but appropriate for any emotion that they wish to express.

Don't worry too much at this stage about trying to recognize the two aspects of Fire. They are difficult to differentiate, even for experienced acupuncturists. Just be aware that there are these two sides to Fire, and give yourself time to see the differences in Fire people.

Having tried to relate what you feel about summer to what the Fire element is about, try and find some video extracts of the people listed below who I think show significant pointers to the Fire element:

- Outer Fire: Tom Cruise, Novak Djokovic, Lang Lang, George Clooney, The Dalai Lama, Archbishop Desmond Tutu, Li Ma, Jackie Chen
- Inner Fire: Tony Blair, Boris Johnson

It does not matter if you have never heard of some of these people. You can still benefit from looking at clips of them. And then look around at friends and family, and think of any of them who make you laugh or who are always trying to please you. Some of you may feel that these people make the atmosphere around them too hot, and you may want to draw back. It is likely to be Metal people who feel this more than any other element. Others may feel that it comforts them and they want to come close, as though to a real fire. These may be Earth or Water people. Earth may enjoy this more than Water people who may start to feel a little anxious if there is too much warmth around. Fire people will enjoy any atmosphere in which there is warmth, and feel very at ease with it. Wood people may quite enjoy it, but not need as much warmth as some of the other elements.

Then add a further exercise. You now have two elements which you have begun to study in depth, Wood and Fire. Take the next important step which is to compare what you have learnt about one element with what you have learnt about the other one. Look at the relevant video extracts of both elements, changing from one to the other, and noting down what differences you think you see. Do the same with people you know who you think may be of these two elements. Compare how you yourself feel when you are happy and your Heart is warm or if you are angry and feel life is not giving you what it should.

Try to pin down what the actual differences are which show that it is a Wood person who is likely to try and push against you or a Fire person who is likely to try and make you smile. Try not to worry if you can't see any differences at first. Never struggle to see what you can't yet see. Let a person come towards you.

If you are lucky, you may be able to transfer the impression one or other famous person has made upon you to somebody you know or to yourself. Maybe a friend or family member is the one that tends to make the room burst out laughing, or another is the one who always likes to tell you what to do. Again, don't try too hard, but let impressions seep into you gradually. If we use our minds too much on trying to disentangle what we are seeing or feeling, we often stifle the emotions we should be experiencing.

Now your studies of the elements are beginning to widen and offer you new insights. By the time you have added the next three elements, your appreciation of their differences will grow as your knowledge increases. Don't try and hurry things by adding another element until you feel you are beginning to have some insight into some of the characteristics of the last element.

B. PRACTICAL WORK

1. Read the 'Alarm points' section in Chapter 4. Learn the alarm points for each official and practise palpating them. Make a card listing the alarm points to go in your little card album.

2. Read the 'Centre pulse' section in Chapter 4. Feel your own centre pulse and see whether you can feel whether it is beating in the centre of the umbilicus. You must be lying down to do this. Feel other people's centre pulse and if the pulse does not feel as if it is in the centre, then start learning how to massage it back into place. You can also try massaging your own centre pulse into position.

3. Pulse-taking notation: Continue increasing the number of pulses you take each day. Now start recording the comparative strengths and weaknesses of the pulses as shown in Chapter 4. The yin and yang officials of one element will nearly always have the same strength, even if they may feel a little different to you. It is very unusual for there to be what we call a 'split pulse' at one pulse position, for example, when the Gall Bladder is -1 and the Liver -2.

   Before writing anything down, take all six pairs of pulses, and then go back and write down what you feel. The strongest pair of pulses should be recorded as +, the weakest as -, and the ones in the middle as a tick ✓.

   Make up a sheet in which you can write down each pulse you take, and fill this in as you take the pulses.

LESSON 4

The Earth element
Akabane test
Touch

A. READING FROM THE HANDBOOK

1. Read the 'Earth element' section in Chapter 2.
2. Learn the list of Earth's characteristics, including:
   * Earth's organs: the Stomach (yang) and the Spleen (yin)
   * Earth's colour, sound, smell and emotion
   * Earth's season and time of day

We have now reached the Earth element, at the centre of the circle of the elements. It can be useful to imagine yourself sitting around a large table laden with food in a warm kitchen, a fire burning in the hearth (here you can think of the Wood and Fire elements helping Earth), and a mother moving between kitchen stove and table feeding her family. The food, the mother and the general sense of cosiness, warmth and being nourished are all images which may help you understand what the Earth element both needs and wants to give. Then think what it would feel like if there was no food on the table, little warmth in the fire and the mother busy doing other things or even not there at all. These are the two extremes of the Earth element which it is worth keeping in mind.

Then look at the following people on video extracts:

Princess Diana, Bill Clinton, Oprah Winfrey, Dawn French, David Cameron, Nigella Lawson, Marilyn Monroe, Dolly Parton

Think now of things that are at the centre, like the hub of a wheel with the spokes turning around it, and then think of what we can see as the centre of the year, its harvest time, as the world gathers in its food to put it in store for the rest of the year. We draw food into ourselves just as nature does in harvest time, and in the same way Earth can be said to pull everything towards itself.

In trying to understand the different elements it helps if we imagine ourselves in the role of each element, by trying to feel inside ourselves what a person must be experiencing who wants the order Wood needs or the love Fire craves, for example. Each element has a particular emotional spectrum which colours their life. Here, with Earth, try to imagine what it must be like to need to draw people towards you, to try to surround yourself with others, to seek nourishment and comfort from them and enclose yourself in their midst. Then add to that the other function of Earth, its reverse side, that of giving out and feeding others, and understand that we can only give out, provide food, if we have something to give.

Then take what you are experiencing inside yourself with you as you look at the video extracts again. Each element expresses its emotional needs in its face in different ways, Fire with its smiling eyes trying to get us to smile, Wood with challenging eyes, and here Earth, not so much with its eyes as with its demanding mouth. The mouth is where we take food in, so look at Earth mouths, and you will see that they are often slightly open, like a baby bird demanding food (what I call the Marilyn Monroe look). It is often to the mouth that our eyes are drawn with Earth people. It is also through the mouth that Earth will show its dissatisfaction, like a child showing it is upset because you have not given it what it wants.

Then see if you can observe some of this kind of Earth need in people you know and in yourself. Do you know somebody who is constantly demanding something from you, wants to be the centre of attention or likes being surrounded by an audience? Do you yourself feel that you are most comfortable in the midst of a group of people? Finally, note how you feel when you are hungry and need food, or are unhappy and would like somebody to look after you. How selfish do these needs make you? And then think of the other side of Earth, and how satisfied you can feel when you make the people around you feel happy and well fed by what you are offering them.

Enjoy being nourished by the Earth element for a little while. Then it will be time to move on to the Metal element, whose needs are quite, quite different. Far from moving forward towards a person, as Earth invites you to do, you are asked to step back and allow Metal to do the work, as you watch it from afar.

B. PRACTICAL WORK

1. Read the 'Akabane test' section in Chapter 4. Practise using the taper in the correct way on yourself first, so that you learn how close to the nail you need to go to warm the nail point. Write down your readings as shown. When you are happy with your technique, start doing the Akabane test on your patients or on volunteers. It is best to do the

procedure with somebody lying down as it is easier to keep the right distance between the taper and the point in this way. You can fold the patient's hands over their stomach to make it quicker to move from left to right hand without going round the couch. If you stand at the end of the couch when you do the feet, you can move easily from left to right foot.

Do at least three tests a week so as to improve your technique.

2. Touch: Whilst doing all the practical exercises, start learning to develop your ability to touch patients in a comforting way, and also to assess how patients respond to your touch. Assessing a patient's response provides a great deal of diagnostic information. We will discuss this in detail in the next lesson, Lesson 5.

Lesson 5

The Metal element
Physical Diagnosis
Importance of touch

A. READING FROM THE HANDBOOK

1. Read the 'Metal element' section in Chapter 2.
2. Learn the list of Metal's characteristics, including:
   - Metal's organs: the Large Intestine (yang) and the Lung (yin)
   - Metal's colour, sound, smell and emotion
   - Metal's season and time of day

The way in which we approach Metal people will be quite different from the way in which we approach Earth. You will need to stand back and watch, and, if you are very observant, you may see that you, in turn, are clearly being watched. And whilst you are being watched, you may feel you are being judged. With this element we move on to much more delicate ground, for we are now in autumn, with none of the fullness and abundance of Fire's summer or Earth's harvest time. Instead, we are in a more rarefied season when the brief flaring of autumn's colours is replaced by the sight of bare branches, the skeletons of trees, announcing the end of the year.

Like its season, Metal sees life in stark outlines, and the need to see things as they truly are makes it a fundamentally serious element. It stands back and observes what life is about, and is most at ease when it is allowed space around it to do this. This need for space will convey itself to others so that, without our being aware of it, we may find ourselves drawing back a little whenever we encounter Metal.

Look carefully at the video extracts of the following people:

Barack Obama, Victoria Beckham, Nelson Mandela, Peter Mandelson, Laurence Olivier, Anthony Hopkins, Ivan Lendl, Daniel Day-Lewis, Tiger Woods

You will see that what all of these people have in common is a sense of detachment and a look of what I call quality. This is something difficult to describe, but easier to see, often in neat clothing and gestures, or a precise, clear way of talking. Victoria Beckham embodies this in the way she dresses, and, interestingly now, in the way she designs clothes. All her clothes have pure, minimalist lines, with the minimum of fuss but the greatest of elegance, and she herself has what I call a typical Metal face, very self-aware and conscious of its own dignity. Metal people often seem to say, 'Look at me, am I not perfect?', and she does this to a very great degree.

Look carefully, too, at Metal eyes. They will appear to you to be far-seeing and observant, often reflecting the sadness which lies at the heart of all that Metal does.

B. PRACTICAL WORK

1. The components of the Physical Diagnosis (Chapter 4): You have now started to practise the following parts of what we call the Physical Diagnosis:

    * Pulse-taking
    * Blood pressure
    * Three jiao
    * Alarm points
    * Centre pulse
    * Akabane test

    Ideally, we should carry all these out the first time we meet our patient. If there is not time to do this, then we need to do them over the first two treatments.

2. The importance of touch: The Physical Diagnosis not only gives you information you need to have, but it also gives you the opportunity to offer your patients something which is often ignored or even discouraged in Western medicine, the gift of your touch. There is an English saying which says that a picture says more than a 1000 words. I think in five element acupuncture we could say that touching our patient in the right way can offer more than 1000 treatments! This is why we use both of our hands to take pulses and to needle, because through our close touch we are already helping to heal our patient's distress.

When I was a student I had to learn how to touch in a way that my patients found comforting, and also to touch different patients in different ways. This is not something that comes naturally to many practitioners, and it took me quite a long time to feel easy with touching patients. When done sensitively it is a great skill which it takes time to learn. Each patient will respond to touch in their own way. Some like a firm touch, others a light touch. We have to be sensitive enough to learn which kind of touch our patients feel comfortable with, and that takes time and practice. With experience you will find that a patient's response to touch can also be used as a further pointer to their element.

There is a practical step you can take here if you suffer from cold hands. Make sure you warm your hands in hot water before approaching a patient, or, as J.R. Worsley told us, just tuck your hands under your armpit for a few moments before going into the practice room. He was a very practical man! The important thing is that your hands should be at blood temperature, and not give your patients a shock.

Lesson 6

The Water Element
Physical Diagnosis

A. READING FROM THE HANDBOOK

1. Read the 'Water element' section in Chapter 2.
2. Read the 'Qualities of the elements' section in Chapter 2.
3. Learn the list of Water's characteristics, including:
   - Water's organs: the Bladder (yang) and the Kidney (yin)
   - Water's colour, sound, smell and emotion
   - Water's season and time of day

Unlike Metal, space is the last thing Water needs, for it likes to fill every nook and cranny as it moves its way forward. We must also think here of nature in winter where everything huddles together to shelter from the cold. Winter is a hidden season, lying beneath a blanket of snow. And Water people always have a hidden side to them.

Within each Water person is an echo of the potential power which water is able to unleash, so that even the gentlest tide can turn the surface of the sea from mirror-like calm into an implacable force swallowing up the land as it rises. You should therefore not be surprised to see how often it is Water people who rise to the top of their profession. If you look carefully at their lives, you will notice that they may often have elbowed other people out of the way without people being aware that this is happening. Their source of power is a hidden one, unlike that of Wood which is displayed quite openly.

The other side to this strength is fear and anxiety. With the Water people I have listed below, look carefully and you may see some of this fear revealing itself in the eyes, which tend either to dart around in a startled way or become too fixed as though trying not to show fear. Water always wants to hide this fear, but may project some of its own anxieties on to those around it. You may therefore find yourself feeling uneasy in its presence without knowing quite why. You may not feel sure what they want of you, and therefore not know how you should react in their presence.

The following are examples of Water people:

David Beckham, Judi Dench, Rowan Atkinson, Gordon Brown, George Osborne, William Hague, Ed Milliband, Andy Murray, Cherie Blair, Roger Federer

With Water we have come full circle on our journey round the elements.

I leave you to think of the gifts that each element bestows upon us:

- The gift of Wood is to start
- The gift of Fire is to relate
- The gift of Earth is to sustain
- The gift of Metal is to extract
- And the gift of Water is the ability to rejoin

B. PRACTICAL WORK

You have now completed all the components of the Physical Diagnosis, and it is time for you to become more used to carrying out a complete Physical Diagnosis on some volunteers or on your patients. See how much time it takes you to do all the different components, and try to speed up so that you can complete all of them within about 30 minutes.

The Physical Diagnosis is carried out as the final part of what we call the Traditional Diagnosis (TD) (Chapter 3). We will be looking in detail at what is needed to carry out a Traditional Diagnosis in the next lesson, Lesson 7.

LESSON 7

The Traditional Diagnosis (TD)
Patient-practitioner relationship
Level of imbalance
Causes of disease

A. READING FROM THE HANDBOOK

1. Read the 'Traditional Diagnosis (TD)' section in Chapter 3.
2. Read the 'Level of imbalance' section in Chapter 3.
3. Read the 'Causes of disease' section in Chapter 3.

In this lesson we move on to look at what can be seen as the most important aspect of five element treatment, our relationship with our patients. If we don't get this right, a patient will not feel that they can trust us enough to tell us about the problems in their life and how they really feel. They may think it is safer to hide their true feelings, and then it will be as though the elements which express these feelings also want to hide from us. If we don't want people to know how we feel, we learn to laugh when we want to cry and hide our fears behind apparent calm. This makes it all the harder to diagnose a patient's guardian element.

The interaction with our patient starts from the first time we meet them, and will gradually build a solid foundation on which we can work. We carry out what we call a Traditional Diagnosis (TD) at this first meeting. There is a checklist of questions in Chapter 3 of the Handbook. You should not go through these questions as if you are asking the patient to fill in a questionnaire, but choose an order which feels natural. Ideally the TD should last 1½–2 hours, and will include the Physical Diagnosis (see Lesson 6). If it is not possible to give a patient this amount of time, the TD should be continued the next time you see the patient until you have all the answers you need to get a good idea of your patient's life, his/her problems and what his/her needs are.

The important thing about a TD is not to spend too much time on concentrating on the physical problems the patient tells you about. Since most patients think acupuncture is only there to treat physical issues, we need to move them gently on to talk about their emotional problems, since we know that these are often the cause of their physical problems. You are not doing a good TD if you find that you have spent most of the time concentrating on physical problems, but have really not got a good understanding of your patient's emotional needs.

B. PRACTICAL WORK

Start preparing to carry out a full Traditional Diagnosis in small stages, using the checklist of questions to guide you. First of all, ask some volunteers to answer some of the questions on the list. Take about half an hour to do this. The volunteer and you should sit next to each other on chairs with a comfortable distance between you, so that it is easy for the volunteer to talk and for you to show your interest in what they are saying. You may be a little embarrassed to ask personal questions when you start, but you will find that you will gradually work out a way of asking these questions which is comfortable for different people. Don't be too critical of yourself. It takes time to relax and not to be self-conscious.

When you feel comfortable doing this, take a little longer to do a TD, and include the other questions. Finally include the Physical Diagnosis. The more you practise these skills, the better you will get at understanding your patients' needs, and this will help point you towards diagnosing their element.

Don't think about elements at all to start with. Just think about learning ways of making your volunteers feel happy to talk to you.

Lesson 8

Sensory and emotional signatures
Training our senses: colour
Acupuncture points

A. READING FROM THE HANDBOOK

1. Read the 'Sensory and emotional signatures' section in Chapter 3.
2. Read the 'Training our senses' section in Chapter 3.
3. Read Chapter 6, 'Acupuncture Points'.
4. Read the 'Command points' section in Chapter 6.

In this lesson we start looking at colour. The colour an element places on the skin colours all the body, and not just that of the face, but since much of the skin is covered by clothing, we tend to look at the face. The simplest way to start trying to detect differences in colour is by standing a small group of people next to each other, with the group taking it in turns to look at the faces of one person after another. Just glance from one person to the next, but don't at this stage try to work out which colour the faces are showing. Just let the colours come towards you. Move the people around a little so that they stand next to different people, and you will probably notice that some of the facial colours seem to change as they move round.

If you are lucky enough to know (or think you know!) what your own guardian element is, place your arm next to the skin of another person (their arm or other part of the body), and compare colours. Colours tend to show themselves most clearly when they are placed next to a colour of a different element.

Don't worry if you can't see any differences in colour yet. It takes a long time, many months or even years, to recognize the colours of the different elements easily, just as it takes time to become sensitive enough to distinguish the sound of voice, smell and, of course, emotion. You will find that changes in patients after treatment can often help your senses develop more sensitivity.

We now look at some of the practicalities of five element treatment procedures. It is important to remember here that all five element treatment is directed at strengthening the guardian element in different ways. To do this, we have to learn to select specific acupuncture points. This lesson will therefore concentrate on the most important grouping of points of all, those called the command points. These are the points which are used both to start and to finish treatment.

J.R. Worsley always said that treatment will be as effective if you use only command points as it will be if you add more complex point selections, 'only it will take a little longer'. For those starting to treat in a five element way for the first time, keep these words of his in mind. Start simple and stay simple, and you won't go wrong. By using command points we are addressing the element we have chosen as guardian element directly and in the simplest way.

One of the first and most important lessons in five element practice is to trust in the power of command points. Good five element practitioners are those who have learnt and understood this basic lesson. In a world which seems to think that the more complex a thing is, the better it must be, learning to rely mainly on command point level treatment is a healthy reminder that what is simple is often the best, and will give practitioners the necessary confidence in their skills.

B. PRACTICAL WORK

1. Collect a small group of people together, and look at the colours of the skin as indicated above. It does not matter if it is always the same people, because you will notice that as your sight becomes more sensitive to colour you will begin to distinguish different types of colour more and more. Try and do this on a regular basis.

2. For all the 12 officials, write an index card listing all the points in the following groups of command points listed in Chapter 6:
    - Source points
    - Element points
    - Horary/seasonal points
    - Junction points
    - Tonification points
    - Sedation points

    If you have not already learnt these points as part of your acupuncture training, gradually learn each group of points so that you don't need to refer to your cards when you are practising.

LESSON 9

Sound of voice
Law of Mother-Child and Sheng and Ke cycles
Tonification, sedation and energy transfers

A. READING FROM THE HANDBOOK

1. Read the 'Law of Mother-Child and Sheng and Ke cycles' section in Chapter 9.
2. Read the 'Energy transfers' section in Chapter 9.

The most frequent form of five element treatment is that of tonification, which means that energy is pushed along a meridian using a specific needling technique which we will look at as part of the practical work in this lesson (see below).

Energy can also be transferred from one element with a relative excess of energy to another with a relative deficiency of energy. Here again, the tonification method of needling is used. Energy can then be passed from a mother element to its child element, using tonification points (see the section on 'Command points' in Lesson 8). It can also be transferred from grandmother element to grandchild element, and in theory from any element to any other element, using the Sheng cycle of energy.

Sedation involves a different needling technique, and is a way of pushing excess energy away to another element. It is used far less often in five element practice, and it is best when you start these lessons to concentrate only on tonification techniques. Do not, therefore, try to learn the principles of doing energy transfers using the sedation method. And at the moment do not try to learn how to do more complex transfers. In practice, we tend to concentrate upon the simplest transfers, those between mother and child element, using tonification points, and just a few from grandmother to grandchild.

B. PRACTICAL WORK

1. Place a few people in a circle and ask each of them to read out the same passage from a book whilst the rest of you close your eyes and just listen. You may be surprised at how different people's voices sound when listened to in this way compared with what you think at first they will sound like. You will slowly begin to hear quite clear differences. At the beginning don't try to work out which elements the sounds of voice are coming from. Instead, just listen to whether the voice is going up or down, whether it is loud or soft, and how it makes you feel inside. Gradually with experience you will learn to associate one type of voice with a specific element. Again, as we said with colour in the last lesson, it takes a long time to recognize a particular tone of voice, so don't be in any hurry, and don't worry if you find the different sounds confusing. You will gradually learn which element the voices belong to as you start treating, and are given other indications of a patient's element.

2. Using a five element chart, try to work out which points you will need to use to take energy from a mother element to its child element for all the five elements using both yin and yang officials of the relevant official. If you find this difficult, try and work in a group with other people. Once you feel confident in finding these points, go on to work out transfers from grandmother to grandchild, remembering that you only use the yin officials for this kind of transfer.

Lesson 10

Training our senses: smell
Aggressive Energy (AE)
Associated Effect Points (AEPs)
Needling techniques

A. READING FROM THE HANDBOOK

1. Read the 'Aggressive Energy' section in Chapter 7.
2. Read the 'Associated Effect Points' section in Chapter 6.
3. Read Chapter 8, 'Treatment Techniques'.
4. Read the 'Needling techniques' section in Chapter 8 (see also needling technique for Aggressive Energy (AE) drain in Chapter 7).

Smell: To develop a sensitive sense of smell you need to get close enough to people to smell their individual body smells. You first have to learn not to be embarrassed at asking fellow-students and friends if you can smell them. The best place to do this is to stand behind them, and smell their neck between the hair line and the shoulder. It is good if the person is hot and therefore sweating quite a lot, but everybody has a particular body smell even when they are not hot. It is useful also to use your own smell to help you. In this case, just put your hand under your armpit and then smell it. You will gradually learn to differentiate smells as you start treating. Very ill people have much stronger smells than healthy people, because their elements are under stress. As patients get more and more healthy, so their body smells change and become less exaggerated.

Just give yourself time to start developing your sense of smell, and, as with the other senses, don't worry if at first you can smell nothing at all.

B. PRACTICAL WORK

1. Practise needling on a potato, an orange or other appropriate object, such as a foam pad, holding the needle as described in Chapter 8. First use the tonification technique described, and then the needle insertion technique for the AE drain described.

2. Make a card listing all the Associated Effect Points (AEPs) (Chapter 6) and AEPs used for AE drain (just the yin AEPs) (Chapter 7).

Lesson 11

Training our senses: emotion
Point selection
Seasonal and daily treatment cycles
Treatment techniques: moxibustion

A. READING FROM THE HANDBOOK

1. Read Chapter 10, 'Point Selection'. Leave the 'Example of point selection for first four treatments' section at the end of the chapter until you have looked at the procedure for clearing possession in Lesson 14.

2. Read the 'Seasonal and daily treatment cycles' section in Chapter 9.

3. Read the 'Sensory and emotional signatures' section in Chapter 3 again.

4. Read the 'Moxibustion techniques' section in Chapter 8.

Emotion: Remind yourself how long it may take to work out which emotion seems to be the one another person is showing. Is it anger (or forcefulness), joy, sympathy (or thoughtfulness), grief or fear? Use every interaction with other people during your daily life to try and work out how they make you feel. This is how you will gradually begin to understand what emotion they are showing, and what emotional reaction in you they are causing. Again, this is a slow process, but you will get quicker at interpreting people's emotions if you practise at every opportunity you can.

B. PRACTICAL WORK

1. Horary times: Write out an index card listing the times at which each official has its greatest energy (horary time).

2. Practise rolling moxa cones, lighting them and removing them quickly until you are confident in your technique. Then start lighting the cones with a taper, first on a dish and then on a volunteer (but not on an acupuncture point!), so that you learn how soon the heat reaches the skin before you remove the cone. The volunteer should tell you immediately they feel the heat, and you should learn to remove the cone very quickly using your thumb and fifth finger. You will quickly

develop some slight scarring on these fingers, and that is why we don't use the second, third or fourth finger, as these are used for pulse-taking and should remain as sensitive as possible. Do this at least once a day.

LESSON 12

The different stages of treatment
Selection of element

A. READING FROM THE HANDBOOK

Read the 'Different stages of treatment' section in Chapter 5.

It is easiest to start treating with five element acupuncture for the first time if you are fortunate to have a qualified acupuncturist to guide you. But if this is not possible, then it is helpful for you to give your first treatment with a small group of other acupuncturists (maximum 2–3) to support you. You should not 'share' the patient as if all of you are that patient's practitioner. In five element acupuncture the important thing, as you know, is to develop a good relationship with your patient, and you can only do this on a one-to-one basis. If other practitioners are in the room with you, they must not interfere with your treatment, but just be there to give you confidence.

The first treatment requires you to take the following steps:

- You must first have carried out a Traditional Diagnosis beforehand (see Lesson 7). You need to do this on your own with your patient to help you establish a good personal relationship from the start. When you have completed the TD as far as you can in one session with your patient, you then have to decide on the guardian element you are choosing to start treatment with.

- You must then select the acupuncture points you will be using for the treatment (see Lessons 13 and 14).

- You should take pulses at each stage of the treatment so that you begin to get used to your patient's pulses. Write down the pulse picture at the start of treatment and at the end of treatment.

Try not to let yourself be influenced by what anybody else thinks your patient's element is; you have to be the one to make the choice. This is the most difficult part of being a five element acupuncturist because nobody can be sure of a patient's element after just a few hours with them. One of the most important qualities of being a five element acupuncturist is learning how to cope with the uncertainty we all feel at the start of treating a patient. The more quickly you get used to this feeling of insecurity, the better! So it is good not to rely on other people's judgement at this stage. Once you have started treating, the results of treatment will help you decide whether you are on the right element or not. Other people's impressions of a patient may be helpful to hear, but they should never override what you are feeling.

Never change the element for at least three treatments, as that will give you time to relax and observe the patient more closely. It's very easy to start hopping from one element to the next, particularly when you first start treating and you are not sure what you are doing. The important thing to remember is that it will be by observing the effects on your patient of treatment concentrated on that one element that will help you decide whether you are on the right element or not.

B. PRACTICAL WORK

Carry out as many Traditional Diagnoses as you can find volunteers prepared to talk to you for two hours or so. Doing a good TD is a skill you have to learn gradually, so the more experience you have the better. Include the Physical Diagnosis at the end of each TD so that you get quicker at carrying out the various tests.

Lesson 13

Possession
Assessing the effects of treatment
Law of Cure

A. READING FROM THE HANDBOOK

1. Read the 'Possession' section in Chapter 7.
2. Read the 'Assessing the effects of treatment' section in Chapter 5.
3. Read the 'Law of Cure' section in Chapter 5.

At the end of each treatment, look at your patient and see if you see any change at all. Sometimes a patient will look happier or calmer, or have a better colour on their face. But don't worry at this stage if you can't see any change. There may be one which you are not sensitive enough yet to see. The important thing to remember is that treatment may take some time to have effect, and that each patient will react differently to treatment.

After the patient has left at the end of each treatment, you should note changes, if any, that you may have observed after treatment. You also need to note down any issues you think you should talk to the patient about at the next treatment, as well as any point suggestions for the next treatment. You should also note any queries you may have about the element you have chosen. See the next lesson, Lesson 14.

B. PRACTICAL WORK

1. Practice looking into a person's eye a few times each week so that you overcome your own hesitation at looking at a person in such an intimate way. The patient must be lying down, as you cannot do this with a person sitting up or standing. Always tell the patient which of your eyes they should look into, and only look into one of the patient's eyes, the one that is closest to you on the couch. Hold the lids firmly apart so that you get a really good look at the pupil to see whether you are able to make contact with their spirit. If a person is not possessed, they will show discomfort and blink or try to look away. A possessed

person will not react in the same way to a long stare into their eye. Their eye often just stays staring at you in an unfocused way.

2. Write out a card with the points for IDs and EDs on them, and the order of insertion. Learn these points.

3. Practise marking out the points for the AE drain and for IDs several times so that you familiarize yourself with the procedure.

LESSON 14

The Law of Husband-Wife
Entry-Exit blocks
Blocks caused by scars
Example of point selection for first four treatments

A. READING FROM THE HANDBOOK

1. Read the 'Law of Husband-Wife' section in Chapter 7.
2. Read the 'Entry-Exit blocks' section in Chapter 7.
3. Read the 'Blocks caused by scars' section in Chapter 7.
4. Read the 'Example of point selection for first four treatments' section in Chapter 10.

The following are the main types of energy blocks:

- Possession (see Lesson 13)
- Aggressive Energy (AE) (see Lesson 10)
- Husband-Wife imbalance (H/W) (this lesson)
- Entry-Exit blocks (this lesson)
- Blocks caused by scars (this lesson)

Read the pages for each of these blocks, and learn the procedures to be used to clear these blocks.

In this section of Chapter 10 you are given an example of the points you can choose at the start of treatment.

B. PRACTICAL WORK

1. Make a card for the points used for clearing a Husband-Wife (H/W) imbalance and Entry-Exit (E/E) blocks. Learn these points and practise marking them up so that you speed up the needling procedure gradually.
2. Continue practising taking pulses on a regular basis (at least 25 a week), and getting used to writing down what you feel. Now you can start differentiating the different pulse qualities a little more. Remember

that a pulse which is -½ is stronger than a much weaker pulse which is -2. Start writing down pulses as shown in Chapter 4. You need to differentiate more and more between different pulse qualities, so that you begin to feel whether energy is blocked in the case of H/W and E/E blocks.

Lesson 15

Windows of the Sky
Further guidelines for selecting points

A. READING FROM THE HANDBOOK

1. Read the 'Windows of the Sky' section in Chapter 6.

2. Read the 'List of my favourite points' section in Chapter 10.

3. Read Chapter 10 of the Handbook again very carefully, paying particular attention to the four different groups of points to be selected at different stages of treatment. Take to heart what I write on the last page of this chapter about the small group of points I myself use.

B. PRACTICAL WORK

1. Make a card for the points for Windows of the Sky, and practise marking these points up.

2. Practise marking up all the non-command points listed in Chapter 10. Look at different patients/volunteers, and try and work out which of the non-command points listed for the first few treatments you think you might choose if you were to treat them.

Lesson 16

Spacing of treatments
Patient's role in treatment

A. READING FROM THE HANDBOOK

1. Read the 'Spacing of treatments' section in Chapter 5.
2. Read the 'Patient's role in treatment' section in Chapter 5.

A great deal of the success of treatment depends upon the elements receiving a gradual and continuing boost to their energy until the patient feels balanced enough either to need no further treatment or to be aware when he/she needs to return for a further boost of energy. Of course, how often a patient comes for treatment will depend on many factors which may make the situation less than ideal, such as the work situation, or living too far from the practitioner for frequent treatments, but it is good to remember that elements need frequent support during the first stages of treatment, and there need to be at least 6–8 weekly treatments to be effective.

It is particularly important, too, that you give the patient enough treatments close enough together for you to be able to assess whether treatment is directed at the right element. At the beginning of treatment we are all unsure about the element, and it is important to see the patient as often as possible to give ourselves time to make a correct diagnosis.

Finally, read the Postscript at the end of the Handbook again to remind yourself that you must not forget that five element acupuncturists are there to help heal a patient's spirit as well as their body.

Conclusion

I have taught you all I can from a distance. Some of you may already have started treating using what you have been learning as you have gone through this course. Others of you may have waited until you have completed the course. All of you will require courage to work on your own in a field of acupuncture which is new to you. It will help you to know that you are following in the footsteps of the pioneers of five element acupuncture's long journey to the West, and in particular J.R. Worsley, whose teachings I am passing on here, and who had to do most of his learning by himself in his own practice room, as there were so few teachers to learn from at that time. If you are working on your own, you, too, will be like a pioneer in the field of five element acupuncture, and are following in this tradition.

If you choose to go on to study and practise five element acupuncture, I am sure that you will gradually feel as privileged as I am at being able to help your patients in so many profound ways. When you are anxious about what you are doing, which is natural as you start to practise, remember that you can never make a patient worse if you treat them in the way I have described in this course. So give yourself plenty of time, try not to hurry, and try not to worry if you can't help some patients. No practitioner can help all the patients who come to him/her. But with practice you will gradually find that you are helping more and more of them to achieve greater balance of body and soul.

The most important lessons you will learn will be those your patients teach you as you start to treat in your own practice, as each treatment becomes a lesson in how to recognize the presence of the elements a little more clearly. The more confident you become in picking up the sensory and emotional signals the elements reveal by their presence, the more quickly you will learn to help your patients. Look closely, too, at all the people around you, at your family, your friends, everybody you meet in the street or at work, and above all at yourself, to help you in your learning.

Finally, I am giving you some tips to help you, a list of dos and don'ts which I have found helpful in my own practice.

1. Keep on repeating this mantra: Don't hurry and don't worry!
2. Remember that the most important aspect of your practice is to feel compassion for your patients and show them your compassion.

Compassion means to 'feel with'. The more you can feel what your patient is feeling, and therefore can understand them, the more quickly you will be able to discover which element is directing their life. Unless we allow our own hearts to resonate with our patient's feelings, we will never understand which of the five elements is their guardian element.

3. The most valuable aspect of the time you spend with your patient is not how long you take to carry out the treatment itself, but the time you give yourselves to get to know and trust each other. Patients won't be counting up how many points you needle, but they will be assessing how interested you are in them and how concerned you are about them.

4. Do not be in a hurry to diagnose the right element! The elements will wait for you to find them, and show their faces more and more clearly with time. And all elements will enjoy the kind of focused attention they receive from simple command point level treatments. If you are not in a hurry, you can relax and learn to get to know your patient better. All of this will give you time to observe whether there has been any change from treatment, and show you whether or not you should continue treating that particular element.

5. Think of each treatment as asking a question of the elements. The practitioner's task is to try to interpret the answers the elements give.

6. Don't confuse the elements by changing from one element to another after only a short time, particularly not in the same treatment, if you are not sure which element you should be treating. Do at least three treatments on any element you choose. If you are treating once a week, then this gives you at least three weeks in which to observe an element's responses. Don't judge any change in your patient simply by using the criteria of physical improvement. Get used to assessing change in the patient as a whole, particularly in the patient's spirit and emotional balance. It is by getting better at noticing what can be even very small changes in a patient's behaviour or physical appearance that we begin to see whether our treatment is directed at the right element.

7. If in doubt, simplify, and do the least number of points possible. Don't judge the success of treatment by the number of points you needle. If you aren't sure where you are going with your treatment, don't add to your confusion by haphazardly adding point to point. Try to clear

CONCLUSION

your mind by just doing one pair of command points, preferably the source points. This helps you focus your attention directly and deeply upon an element. Then let the elements answer you.

8. Don't spend too long trying to diagnose the blocks, such as possession, Husband/Wife or Entry-Exit blocks. They are much more difficult to diagnose than you may think. It doesn't matter if you miss them to start with. They become more and more obvious the longer they remain untreated. An expert practitioner may see them straightaway; a less experienced practitioner will inevitably take longer to recognize them. There is a risk that a newly qualified practitioner will over-diagnose blocks because of the excitement of doing them.

9. Don't think that your patient is necessarily expecting a quick fix. Patients are usually only too happy to give the practitioner all the time they need. It is usually you are who are in more of a hurry than your patient. Patients appreciate the care and deep concern their practitioner shows them, and return again and again for that. They are delighted that you are so interested in helping them, compared with the impersonal approach of a doctor's surgery or hospital waiting room.

And now I wish you all the courage to explore the mysterious world of the elements in a healthy spirit of adventure.

Printed in Great Britain
by Amazon